MANTALK

Tips from the Pros on Good Looks,
Good Health, and Maintaining
Your Competitive Edge

Elliot W. Jacobs, MD, FACS

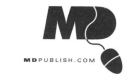

MDPUBLISH.COM

DISCLAIMER

The information contained in this book represents the opinions of the author and should by no means be construed as a substitute for the advice of a qualified medical professional. The information contained in this book is for general reference and is intended to offer the user general information of interest. The information is not intended to replace or serve as a substitute for any medical or professional consultation or service. Certain content may represent the opinions of Elliot Jacobs MD, FACS based on his training, experience, and observations; other physicians may have differing opinions.

All information is provided "as is" and "as available" without warranties of any kind, expressed or implied, including: accuracy, timeliness, and completeness. In no instance should a user attempt to diagnose a medical condition or determine appropriate treatment based on the information contained in this book. If you are experiencing any sort of medical problem or are considering cosmetic or reconstructive surgery, you should base any and all decisions only on the advice of your personal physician who examined you and entered into a physician-patient relationship with you.

This book is designed to provide information of a general nature about cosmetic procedures. The information is provided with the understanding that the author and publisher are not engaged in rendering any form of medical advice, professional services, or recommendations. Any information contained herein should not be considered a substitute for medical advice provided person-to-person and/or in the context of a professional treatment relationship by qualified physician, surgeon, dentist, and/or other appropriate healthcare professional to address your individual medical needs. Your particular facts and circumstances will determine the treatment that is most appropriate to you. Consult your own physician and/or other appropriate healthcare professional on specific medical questions, including matters requiring diagnosis, treatment, therapy, or medical attention. Any use of the information contained within is solely at your own risk. MDPress, Inc. assumes no liability or responsibility for any claims, actions, or damages resulting from information provided in the context contained herein.

ISBN-13: 978-0-9748997-6-3
ISBN-10: 0-9748997-6-3

Printed in the United States of America.

Book design by StarGraphics Studio

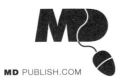

MD PUBLISH.COM   350 Fifth Avenue, Suite 7619 | New York, New York 10118

About the Author

Elliot William Jacobs, MD received his undergraduate education from Queens College and his medical degree from Mount Sinai School of Medicine in New York City. He completed his internship and residency in general surgery at Mount Sinai Hospital and then continued at Mount Sinai as resident and chief resident in plastic surgery.

Dr. Jacobs is certified by the National Board of Medical Examiners and the American Board of Plastic Surgery. He is a fellow of both the American College of Surgeons and the International College of Surgeons. He is a member of the American Society of Plastic Surgeons, the American Society for Aesthetic Plastic Surgery, and Mensa.

Dr. Jacobs is licensed to practice medicine in New York, New Jersey, California, and the Bahamas. He serves as an honorary police surgeon for the New York City Police Department and as a consultant in plastic surgery to the United Nations. He is on the attending staff of several hospitals in Manhattan and New Jersey.

Dr. Jacobs has written on many aspects of plastic surgery in professional literature and has lectured to both professional and lay groups around the world. He has been featured in the national and local media including MTV, ABC *20/20*, *Discovery Health*, *The David Letterman Show*, *The Joan Rivers Show*, and many others.

Acknowledgements

I am most grateful for the contributions of Marc Lowenberg, DDS; Max Gomez, Ph.D; Allen Greenbaum, MD; Howard Murad, MD; Frederic Fekkai, David Finley and Oz Garcia, all of whose expertise has added immeasurably to the contents of this book. A special thank you to Dr. Max Gomez, Dr. Martin Lubin, Dr. Perry Robins, and Frederic Fekkai for your kind words of praise. And a deep appreciation to the team of MDPublish, who have helped and guided me throughout the development of this book, from initial idea to completed manuscript. Most of all, to my beautiful Leigh, whose love, patience, and encouragement have been a blessing to my life.

*To Leigh and Ben, for all your love,
inspiration and encouragement.*

*To my staff, who have worked tirelessly
for me, my patients, and this book.*

*To my teachers and colleagues, who have
taught me with patience and understanding.*

*And to my patients, who present
daily challenges to my skills and a mandate
to become an even better surgeon
with every operation performed.*

Contents

Foreword

It is a common stereotype that men do not like asking for directions. Personally, I hate getting lost and have no problem asking for directions, but there are more than enough men who don't ask for help to keep the image alive. Not only is this true when traveling, but in other aspects of our lives as well.

As a medical reporter for more than twenty-five years I have found that men are not all that great at taking care of their health, especially if it involves asking for information (kind of like asking for directions). I have also found that men rely on women to be their source for most health-care information

So when it comes to something as personal as plastic surgery, where are men going to turn for information? The women in their lives? Unlikely. They are reluctant to ask in the first place and probably do not want to seem vain. And how many men are going to ask another man for a referral to a plastic surgeon? Not many. Besides, men are tacticians, and before anyone puts a scalpel near our faces, we want to do the research ourselves to be sure that the surgeon knows what he or she is doing. But most of us do not have the time to make this a lifelong pursuit.

This is why *MANTALK* by Dr. Elliot W. Jacobs is such an important book. It is a cosmetic surgery, skincare, and grooming navigation system written by a man for men. It covers the bevy of treatments and procedures in the way men are used to communicating. It is straightforward and concise and very cutting edge. And it is a not a hard sell for going under the knife. On the contrary, all the options are revealed in detail, from Botox® injections to hair removal lasers and other non-surgical innovations. *MANTALK* also expands its scope to include the realms of nutrition, fitness, dentistry, haircare and laser vision correction for today's man.

This is what I would expect from Dr. Jacobs, a veteran New York plastic surgeon, whom I have known for more than a decade. His intelligence, experience, and ability to articulate medical information in layman's terms are what set him apart. Dr. Jacobs is widely recognized for bringing the sensitive issue of gynecomastia, the abnormal enlargement of the male breast, out of the closet and into public discourse. He is an innovator in the field, and extremely selective about the surgeries he offers to his male patients to insure a high rate of satisfaction. In short, he "gets" it.

No matter what treatments, procedures, or surgeries you might be considering to improve your looks, *MANTALK* gives you the straight talk you need to actually take the plunge.

—Max Gomez, Ph.D
Medical Correspondent, WNBC-TV

Introduction

MAN IN THE MIRROR

"You can't help getting older, but you don't have to get old."

—**George Burns**

The open expression of male vanity is undoubtedly on the rise. The male grooming market has been cited as an industry of $3.5 billion and growing, especially among graying baby boomers and hip generation X-ers. Men are spending heavily on grooming products, hair restoration, teeth whitening, and cosmetic surgery in the relentless pursuit of youth and perfection. Let us face it: men are now competing with other men, as well as with women, who have been bred for centuries to learn how to take care of themselves. With pretty boy role models like Ben Affleck and Brad Pitt, the "average Joe" may need a head-to-toe makeover to keep up.

Man's perpetual quest for self-improvement has now stretched far beyond a mere desire to acquire material possessions. Men are also seeking ways to improve their health and transform their physical appearance. Although every age group has concerns about body image, those most vulnerable are Americans crossing the threshold into middle age and beyond, otherwise known as the boomers.

Men have long been clued into the importance of the "dress for success" motto in order to maintain their edge. Image enhancing systems, gadgets, and treatments are the next logical step. Whereas some men are still fighting it kicking and screaming, others have come to embrace looking good as a status symbol that goes with the Breitling Chronograph and the Gucci laptop case. There was a time when caring too much about his looks made a man seem feminine or vain. Today it comes with the territory—success means never have to apologize for looking after yourself.

As concerns about personal appearance have become a common topic of conversation, the skincare industry has responded with a host of new products designed especially for men. This demand can be traced to changes in men's lifestyles, and consumer behavior beginning with the economic boom of the 1980s and through the dotcom wave of the 1990s. During this time men increasingly moved away from traditional labor professions and into the office, where they have the time, money, and need to care for their appearance. As men saw success in both their professional and social lives, they reaped the benefits of spending more time and money on their personal appearance. Aided by an onslaught of men's magazines—which avidly embrace a well-groomed man—traditional products such as shaving cream, razors, deodorants, colognes, and hair styling products have become more appealing and varied. This awareness has translated into an expanded male-hygiene market as well as acceptance and desire among men to improve what nature and genetics gave them through cosmetic surgery.

In the past several years, the emerging metrosexual has opened a new conversation about men's grooming. Coined by writer Mark Simpson, the term describes an urban male with a strong aesthetic sense who freely and openly spends time and money on his appearance and lifestyle. As the metrosexual phenomenon has made it hip and acceptable for men to indulge in grooming routines, sales for "beauty" products geared toward men have skyrocketed. Sales of male-oriented products have grown twice as fast as those of female-oriented products.

I have noticed a worldwide boom in men secretly having cosmetic enhancements. In my practice on New York's Park Avenue, we are seeing about 35 percent men, and that number is growing. And it is not just actors and news anchors anymore. Past a certain age, men start to see things they do not like in the mirror, and they are making the decision to do something about it.

I have maintained a private cosmetic surgery practice in New York since 1979. My practice encompasses a full range of aesthetic surgery, including all facial, breast, and body procedures for men and women. The evolution of *MANTALK* is a culmination of the direction my private cosmetic surgery practice has taken over the past several years. *MANTALK* is based on the questions and concerns that my male patients, colleagues, and friends deal with every day. I have assembled some key experts in their fields to enhance the information provided in this innovative book for men. The irony is that many of my female patients, along with the wives and partners of my own circle of acquaintances, are eagerly awaiting this book, too. They see the void on the market for credible, healthy aging advice for men about what works and what makes sense. They want practical tips for staying fit, vigorous, and liking what you see in the bathroom mirror while you are shaving. I hope you enjoy this book as much as we have enjoyed bringing the components together for you into one volume.

CHAPTER 1

The Aging Man

*Despite what you might think,
no two men age at the same rate.*

As we age, we go through gradual states of change. With each passing year our skin loses its ruddiness, structure, and youthful resiliency. Aging is genetically programmed through biochemical changes in collagen and elastin, the connective tissues that give the skin its firmness and elasticity. Because every man's genetic program is individual, the loss of skin firmness and elasticity occur at different rates and times. As early as age thirty-five the skin begins a slow, gradual descent. By age sixty, the skin visibly sags. Sagging is especially noticeable on the face because it endures more environmental and UV damage. As the skin loses its structure and elasticity, it can no longer fight the effects of gravity. A lifetime of repeated pulling by the muscles under the skin, coupled with damage from smoking, alcohol and environmental exposure, play a role in the formation of wrinkles.

Genetically programmed aging occurs alongside the process of photoaging—the effects of chronic and excessive sun exposure on the skin. Photoaging is responsible for as much as 90 percent of age-associated changes in the skin's appearance, such as mottled pigmentation, surface roughness, fine wrinkles that disappear when stretched, brown spots on the hands, and dilated blood vessels. Sun damage is cumulative. To reduce the effects of chronological and photoaging, sun exposure and tanning must be effectively eliminated, and a comprehensive program combining state-of-the-art skincare with clinical treatment solutions should be implemented. There is no magic bullet.

MALE VS FEMALE AGING

The aging process differs significantly between male and female skin. In men, each year the skin gradually thins at the rate of approximately 1 percent per year. In women, however, the thickness of the skin remains surprisingly constant until menopause, after which there is a significant and sometimes dramatic thinning with age. This difference in skin thickness is attributed to the relationship between skin thickness and collagen content. While collagen content in both sexes decreases with age, it does so at different rates. As women age, they may look older than men of the same age and similar amounts of sun exposure because their skin initially has a lower collagen content. Varying collagen contents may also be related to the difference in hormone production between men and women. Because estrogen and androgen output from the ovaries and adrenal glands decreases after menopause, collagen synthesis and repair in women go down as well. The decline of estrogen production coupled with photoaging can dramatically increase the apparent age of a menopausal woman. Men, on the other hand, do not experience significant declines in estrogen, so they do not appear to age as rapidly as women.

Although skin elasticity decreases with age in everyone, the effect is more pronounced in women than in men. As skin loses its elasticity, it appears fragile because it lacks deep, solidly connected cells that are protected by natural oils, which also decline with age. The decline of these natural oils, however, is more rapid in women than men.

HOW MEN AGE		
AGE	APPEARANCE	FUNCTION
<18	Nearly perfect skin Smooth texture, small pores	Excellent repair capabilities Low productivity of oil Good skin hydration
18–25	Acne key factor in surface texture Fine lines start to appear, pore size increases	High productivity of oil Drop in dermal repair, immune system, and collagen synthesis Strong cohesion between skin layers and rapid cell turnover Small drop in skin hydration, noticed particularly in winter
25–45	More fine lines and appearance of first wrinkles Early signs of sagging near the eye Some loss of elasticity Adult acne	Moderate decrease in dermal repair, less collagen, increase in damaged connective tissue Noticeable drop in skin hydration
45–55	More wrinkles, rough texture Sallow yellow color Pores and age spots enlarge Sagging near eyes and cheeks	Significant decrease in dermal repair and immune system Continued dermal degradation Cohesion between skin layers continues to decline Thinning of skin and deep tissues Skin tends to be dry
55+	Wrinkles and fine lines in abundance Uneven color, pigmentation Sagging worsens Dark circles under the eye	Comprised dermal repair, abundance of damaged connective tissue Low production of collagen and oil Increased local over-production of melanin

WRINKLE REDUCTION

Fine lines are due to the breakdown of collagen and elastin fibers over time. This is exacerbated by the sun damage that men accumulate over the years. Deep wrinkles are typically associated with the constant action of musculature below the skin's surface. Over time, facial expression muscles will thicken the muscle, just like building up your biceps. Deep wrinkle lines may be present on a persistent basis (static wrinkles seen with the face at rest), or may be seen only when those muscles are used (dynamic wrinkles). For example, some men's crow's feet are only obvious when they smile because their cheeks come up, or their frown lines may be evident only when they frown.

Therapy for wrinkles is aimed at correcting many issues. Some are preventative, others are restorative. Sun-damaged skin is characterized by a weakening of supporting collagen and elastin fibers caused by a reduction in collagen production. The key to maintaining your skin is to keep it taught, with good structure and elasticity. Cosmetic surgery, such as a facelift, is most effective for deep wrinkles and sagging skin in the lower face. It is somewhat effective in the middle face, yet not very effective for the upper face.

Classifying Wrinkles

- **Crinkle-type wrinkles**—Fine wrinkles formed around folded skin; generally seen in the elderly and men with sun damage.

- **Glyphic wrinkle**—A crisscross pattern that makes a diamond shape; usually found on the cheeks, neck, and hands.

- **Deep wrinkles**—A major line or deep grooves; usually long and straight.

Fat Migration

As you turn the corner from the thirties to the forties, one of the first signs of aging is the loss of soft, round, cherubic fullness. As you get older, you actually need all the fat you can get in your face, while it becomes harder to keep it off your body. Men tend to gain weight as they grow older. The little fat pad under the chin and pouches along the jaw line start to expand. As the natural fat of your face changes shape, hollows start to show up around the eyelids, the middle of the cheeks, and around the mouth. The fatty layer on the backs of the hands, the neck, and the face becomes noticeably thinner. This leads to more noticeable blood vessels on the hands. Fat pads moving south below the eyes exacerbate the appearance of dark circles, and the overall thinning of the skin allows for increased fragility. The disappearance of facial fat also exacerbates some of the deeper wrinkling changes along the jawline and around the mouth.

Muscle Relaxing

Below the skin layer lies the fat and beneath that is muscle. Deep wrinkles are due to the build-up of muscles in areas of overused facial expressions, such as smiling or frowning. The same can be said of the deep lines that form around the mouth, sometimes called smoker's lines. Chronic puckering of the mouth—particularly if there is additional sun damage—may lead to the formation of deep creases and folds which will require different therapy than treatments for finer lines associated with damage within the dermis or deeper tissue.

Non-Surgical Age Management

Today's man has embraced the concept of having multiple non-invasive, non-surgical treatments for lines, creases, and folds.

Skin rejuvenation is not about looking thirty-five when you turn fifty. Rather, it is about choosing a reasonable approach to caring for your skin, maintaining its health, and moisturizing to keep it looking healthy.

Making the most of what science and technology have to offer, the war against wrinkles is being fought with an arsenal of fillers and injectable substances. In my practice, the most popular non-surgical treatments for men are Botox® and dermal fillers such as Radiesse®, Sculptra®, and Restylane®. These treatments have the advantage of being safe, effective, affordable, and quick. Many of my male patients schedule a procedure before an early meeting, at the end of the workday, or during lunch, since there is little or no downtime.

My Philosophy

The key to anti-aging is maintenance. Compare it to working out. You cannot just go to the gym once; you have to keep going to maintain the benefits of a fitness program.

I am a big advocate of doing everything one can to prevent wrinkles, rather than waiting to correct wrinkles once they have appeared. I routinely recommend to my patients—especially the younger ones—to begin with smaller, less-invasive procedures and earlier surgery. Not everyone wants to have a facelift, even if we will all ultimately benefit from surgery to correct skin laxity and sagging. Many of my male patients prefer to concentrate on non-surgical, minimally invasive procedures combined with active skincare to forestall the need for surgery until later.

CHAPTER 2

Zone Specific Surgery

Men and women both covet youth;
men just know how far to go to get it.

Aesthetic plastic surgery for men is growing exponentially around the world. Statistics indicate that men account for about 20 percent of all the procedures done in the world's capitols, and 30 percent in Brazil. Most plastic surgeons now feature the most recent *Sports Illustrated* and *Esquire*, along with *Vogue* and *Allure* in their waiting rooms.

But the bodies, goals, and temperaments of men are different from those of women. Men are impatient with long recovery periods and prefer to have procedures that do not require maintenance. Men need techniques that will ensure a masculine look with less recovery time. They are also not into pain.

SUBTLE SURGERY

Subtle surgery does not draw attention to itself but rather it draws attention to YOU.

The goal of modern cosmetic surgery, especially for men, is what I call *subtle surgery*. It enhances what nature gave the individual and leaves him looking refreshed, less tired, and more energized without any of the telltale signs of surgery that should always be avoided, such as slanted, hollow eyes and pulled cheeks. Conservative surgery should be the mantra for male cosmetic surgery. Techniques have improved so tremendously that we can now offer out patient surgery with minimal downtime. I often customize a procedure to a specific zone of the face or neck. For example, most men tend to be bothered more by the aging changes that appear in the lower face and neck (called a "turkey gobbler") rather than the upper face and brow.

I routinely perform a neck lift in men. It tightens the musculature of the neck, reduces excess fat under the chin and jawline, and tightens sagging skin to eliminate jowls. The incision is carefully designed to follow the anatomy of the ear and curls around the earlobe without disrupting the hairline. On younger men with thicker and more elastic skin, I often use liposuction alone to sculpt the neck and jawline area. A minimally invasive Contour Threadlift™ combined with liposuction can firm and tighten neck skin without making any major incisions. Occasionally, if the chin is receding, I may also add a chin implant at the same time to further enhance the jaw line. This procedure can take years off a man's appearance with minimal recovery and discomfort.

GETTING READY FOR COSMETIC SURGERY

Cosmetic surgery is real surgery. Any time I pick up a scalpel, it is indeed real surgery. As with any surgery, there are risks and the results are long lasting so it is extremely important to do your research. If you are well-informed, you will have a much better working relationship with your surgeon. By establishing a good rapport with your surgeon, you can develop an approach together that will produce the results that you want. Most of all, you want a doctor who is highly experienced and who will customize a procedure for you based on your skin or body type, your age, your medical history, the best technology available, and your individual specifications. I never perform the identical procedure on every patient. Every man has a different bone structure, skin quality, and goal so I tailor my approach to the individual.

GETTING BACK TO WORK

In my experience, the hardest aspect of undergoing surgery for men is the recovery. Therefore, we devote special care and attention to speeding up the healing process so men can get back to their busy lives as quickly as possible.

MALE TALE: Jack, an investment banker in his 50s, scheduled his mid-facelift around a lull in his otherwise hectic work life. Like most men, he did not tell anyone that he was having a little work done. The day before he was coming in for surgery, his boss (a young buck in his late 30s) called an emergency meeting for later that week. Jack started to panic. He called my office and asked me what he should do. I suggested that he arrange to conference into the meeting from his house in East Hampton and use a speaker phone to avoid disturbing the area around his ears. His surgery was done on a Monday, and by that Thursday morning, he was able to participate in the meeting electronically without any problem. By the following week, he was back in action, as good as new but looking even better.

Tissue Glue

Some swelling and bruising are to be expected after surgery, but today's methods are designed to minimize recovery. Although fibrin sealant or "tissue glue" has been used in surgery for more than twenty years, it is relatively new to plastic surgery. Fibrin glues the wound edges together and acts as a growth hormone, both of which allow healing to begin promptly. With a fibrin sealant, less swelling and bruising are seen post-op, and drains and bulky dressings are no longer needed.

CHAPTER 3

About Face

*Although the basic concepts of a facelift
are the same for men and women, I favor
a customized approach to facial rejuvenation.*

Men seeking to correct the signs of facial aging present unique challenges for surgeons, often requiring modifications to surgical techniques used for female patients. When men do have facelifts, their thicker skin requires a unique procedure: less pulling of the skin itself, which tends to become overly thin when pulled, and more work tightening the deeper tissues of the face.

In men, a facelift involving significant correction of the neck requires incisions in front of and behind the ear. Plastic surgeons have developed various techniques for hiding these incisions, often within natural lines and creases. While women's hairstyles generally make it easier to conceal the incisions, it is understandable that men are particularly concerned with avoiding any telltale or visible scarring in the hairless area in front of the ear.

With changing standards of aesthetics of the male face, more men are seeking the benefits of facial cosmetic surgery procedures. Although the concept of a facelift in men is basically the same as in women, I tailor my approach to sharpen the angular structures of the jaw, neck, and chin, with less emphasis on superficial lines, wrinkles, and creases. Although facelift and necklift methods will restore facial contours, they will not address the texture or quality of the skin, which can be improved by resurfacing techniques. The appearance of fresher and crisper contours leads to a more relaxed look without any distortion.

THE MID-FACE LIFT

Early signs of aging include creases and deep folds around the mouth and also from the side of the nose to the outer corners of the mouth. In men, due to thicker skin, these show up perhaps in their early to mid-fifties, slightly later than with women. The central oval of the mid-face has traditionally been the most difficult area to improve through surgery. I favor the mid-facelift technique to address many of these problems. It is performed through the classic lower eyelid incision and allows me to rejuvenate the triangle between the inner and outer corners of the eye and the corner of the mouth. This technique gently lifts the tissues of the mid-face and elevates the fat and skin tissue to the original position it occupied when a man was in his early thirties.

With the mid-facelift procedure that I have developed, the fat bags under the eyelids are eliminated, nose-to-mouth creases are softened, and the lid/cheek junction line is smoothed to create a more youthful appearance.

The Contour Threadlift™

Every man I know, including myself, has at one time looked in a mirror, lifted the facial skin and wished it would stay right there. Now it is possible to do just that with a minimally invasive technique which takes less than an hour to perform. The Contour Threadlift™ is an ideal procedure for male patients who are unwilling to undergo invasive surgery to look younger.

As aging progresses, our face and neck skin and soft tissues begin an inexorable drift downwards due to the loss of collagen and elasticity, exposure to the elements, gravity and our own unique genetic makeup. Smoking only adds to the problem. Deepening creases, folds, and loose skin are the result. These changes can be seen as early as the mid-thirties. As much as we pull the skin upwards in the mirror, we may also wonder if we are too young for a conventional "facelift."

The Contour Threadlift™, is a safe and effective procedure, performed under local anesthesia and mild sedation, can elevate the eyebrows (or correct asymmetric eyebrows), the cheeks and jowls and tighten lax neck skin. It involves the placement of multiple, long-lasting "barbed" sutures through tiny incisions in the scalp or ear. The tiny bristles on each suture will open like multiple mini-umbrellas when placed into tissue and then catch and hold the tissue while the suture is tightened. The sutures themselves are clear and colorless and have been safely used in patients for many years. Once the sutures are placed, the body will generate new collagen around each "thread" to hold it in place. The result is a natural, soft, and gentle elevation of the tissues without major surgery.

The average procedure will take about an hour or less to perform. Afterwards treatment with cold compresses will help to minimize any swelling and bruising. It usually takes between three to seven days to see the final result. The post-treatment discomfort is relatively minimal. Most of my male patients can be seen in public within a few days after the procedure but strenuous activity should be avoided for seven to ten days.

Physicians' experiences have shown results that endure for three years or longer, depending on the age of the patient at the time of the procedure and the number of threads utilized. The real advantage of a Contour Threadlift™ is that if necessary, the threads can be tightened or additional threads may be inserted to provide more lift later on. In addition, the results of a Contour Threadlift™ can always be refined and improved by combining it with other non-surgical procedures including peels, lasers, and fillers such as Restylane® and Botox®. We can always do a conventional facelift at a later date if desired.

Which men are the best candidates for this procedure?

The Contour Threadlift™ can be performed on men in their forties to their sixties. Sometimes a simple Restylane® treatment will accomplish what men are looking for, and in other cases, only a formal face- and neck-lift will do. In many cases, a Contour Threadlift™ appeals to a man who fears surgery and is merely seeking a subtle lifting effect without the telltale signs of having had anything done. I have been very pleased with the results I can achieve with this procedure and am pleased to offer it to my patients.

CHAPTER 4

Open Your Eyes

The surgeon who applies the same aesthetic criteria to both men and women is guilty of an error in aesthetic judgment.

The eyelids in men age in several ways. Eyelid skin lacks oil content, which leaves it more prone to wrinkling. Droopy eyelids or puffy lower eyelids often run in families and are equally common in men and women. At first, bags or sagging may be most noticeable when you are particularly tired, and the signs become increasingly visible all the time. Eyelid skin thins and stretches with time, muscles weaken, and fat that cushions the eyeball moves forward under the eyes. Puffiness results when a fat pad that cushions the eye begins to push against weakened tissues and then protrudes outward, thereby forming a "bag." Sagging upper eyelids may result in hooding, where upper lids become heavier and fuller. Droopy eyebrows may further accentuate the excessive upper eyelid skin.

MALE EYE AESTHETICS

In my view, a conservative approach is the essence of appropriate eyelid surgery for men. Eyelid surgery should never compromise the functional elements of the eyelids for the sake of aesthetics. I can remove the excess fat and drooping skin of the upper eyelids, minimize bags under the eyes, and tighten lower eyelid skin. More minimally invasive techniques such as fat removal from the lower eyelids will often produce enough improvement as a solo procedure in younger men with good skin tone. In older patients, I may opt to do skin excision and/or muscle tightening to achieve an optimum effect. The result is a restored and more rested appearance without changing the shape or size of the eyes and without an excessively tight look.

EYELID REJUVENATION

While the techniques for performing cosmetic eyelid surgery on a man are fundamentally the same as those used on a woman, there are several factors that men should be aware of when considering eyelid surgery. First, since men do not wear eye makeup and concealer, the procedure must reflect this. Externals scars will be more visible, especially during the early healing process. Aesthetically, women desire a high and deep upper eyelid crease as the final result from eyelid surgery to give themselves a defined platform that can be enhanced with makeup. Because men do not wear eye makeup, this result on men is undesirable and should be avoided. Sometimes I will deliberately leave some skin so it looks natural.

In lower eyelid surgery, transconjunctival lower blepharoplasty is often performed, since the incision must be made very carefully to avoid having to conceal a scar with cosmetics.

Because men want to preserve their rugged exterior and to avoid a feminizing look, the final result should appear as natural as possible, which often means a certain degree of intentional under correction. Most men wish to look "refreshed" rather than "rejuvenated"; in other words, more energetic rather than simply younger or "done."

MALE TALE: Harris is a 45-year-old matrimonial attorney with his own law firm. Every morning at 7 A.M. he hits the ground running. He works out three times a week at the gym in his office building, and keeps himself in good shape, but his wife says he looks tired all the time. "I guess I look tired because I am tired," says Harris, "but if I keep this up, I'm going to look like my own father pretty soon." So Harris formulated a plan of action. He decided to get rid of the fat bags under his eyes once and for all. We removed the excess fat under Harris' eyes using a transconjunctival approach (inside the lower eyelid), which avoids any visible scar. He was back in divorce court in five days with a slight bruise under his right eye. "The judge just assumed that an irate husband took a swing at me," says Harris.

LIFTING HEAVY BROWS

Men too are becoming increasingly concerned about the appearance of their eyelid and eyebrow region and the message it may depict. For a number of reasons, men are now more likely to consider eyelid or eyebrow rejuvenation surgery in order to eliminate the tired look associated with heavy lids or lateral hooding. Men are more prone to consider cosmetic surgery when the initial evaluation is coupled with a functional concern. While men seek information about cosmetic surgery to correct a physical defect or functional concern, this initial dialogue then opens the door to discussion about other concerns. For instance, the male patient who initially asks about a visual field defect caused by excessive upper eyelid skin may often be willing to discuss further aesthetic features of eyelid and eyebrow abnormalities.

MALE VS FEMALE FACIAL AESTHETICS

In principle, the concept of lifting the eyebrows may be quite similar between women and men. In practice, however, there are quite a number of differences. Women, because of plucking, waxing, and coloring their eyebrows, are generally much more aware of the position of their eyebrows and how the eyebrow effects facial expression. Men are usually less aware of how the eyebrows may contribute to what they perceive as a tired look. Women seem to grasp intuitively the concept of brow lifting, possibly because they have so often stimulated the "look" by holding their brows up while standing in front of a mirror. Men, in general, are initially surprised by the suggestion of a brow lift as a solution. Most men expect that only a simple procedure is necessary and are often ill-prepared for the discussion about brow lift techniques. A brow-lift is perceived by men as a much bigger ordeal, and some may even find it threatening.

Once men have grasped the concept of a brow lift, the differences between male and female aesthetics can be outlined and an appropriate surgical plan designed to achieve an aesthetically pleasing result. Many features of the upper face convey the physical differences between men and women. The male eyebrow generally sits lower on the brow and takes on an almost horizontal shape with less arch. A high-arched eyebrow is a distinctly feminine characteristic that appears unusual and unnatural on the male face.

Creases across the forehead and frown lines between the eyebrows are considered aging and objectionable on women but can imply strength, power, and wisdom on men. Culturally, it seems more acceptable and expected that a man's face has lines and furrows. These character lines are perceived in many cases to make a man look more distinguished—a perception that most men want to preserve because many cultures and many men admire and even enjoy these creases and lines. Surgery can soften these features on men without eliminating them entirely.

Distinct differences also exist between men and women in the upper eyelid. The male upper lid is decidedly fuller, and it sometimes appears more masculine if slightly redundant. This is yet another reason not to lift the male brow too high. Men are primarily concerned with lateral brow hooding and redundant upper eyelid skin.

BROW PEXY

The brow pexy is an operation that is used to reposition the eyebrows. It improves the appearance of the brows and can make the eyes look less crowded, larger, and more open. Brow pexy is usually done along with a facelift or eyelid procedure but can be performed as a stand alone procedure. In a suspension brow lift, two to four small incisions are made in each eyebrow. They extend into the upper temporal area and are made for needle entry. The surgeon will place hidden permanent sutures to produce the lift. The scars are very small, and the procedure can be repeated if needed. This technique is especially good for men because it avoids any lengthy incisions in the hairline. For women with low eyebrows and a high hairline, it is a possible alternative to more classic brow lift procedures.

FOREHEAD CREASES

The corrugator muscle is the muscle that creates vertical wrinkles between the eyebrows (the "worry lines"), making a person appear to be scowling or angry. Whereas botulinum toxin injections can effectively weaken the corrugator muscle for three to four months, thereby reducing the appearance of lines and wrinkles, the surgical division of the muscle permanently weakens it. This can be done through either a brow lift approach or, more commonly, via the upper eyelid in conjunction with upper eyelid blepharoplasty. A small incision is made on the inner corner or the edge of each eyebrow, and the corrugator muscle is severed on both sides. This procedure may be performed under local anesthesia and is often combined with other facial procedures. In many cases, injections of botulinum toxin may effectively soften forehead creases to avoid the need for surgery. However, as the effects last three to four months on average, this would have to be repeated frequently, which many men do not want.

SEEING CLEARLY

To see clearly, the cornea and the lens must bend—or refract—light rays so they focus on the retina—a layer of light-sensing cells that line the back wall of the eye. The retina converts the light rays into impulses that are sent to the brain, where they are recognized as images. If the light rays do not focus on the retina, the image you see is blurry. This is called a refractive error. Glasses, contacts, and refractive surgery attempt to reduce these errors by making light rays focus on the retina.

Refractive errors are caused by an imperfectly shaped eyeball, cornea, or lens and are of three basic types:

- **Myopia**—nearsightedness; only nearby objects are clear
- **Hyperopia**—farsightedness; only objects far away are clear
- **Astigmatism**—images are blurred at a distance and when near

Presbyopia, also known as the aging eye, usually occurs between ages forty and fifty and can be corrected with bifocals or reading glasses. Some signs of presbyopia include a tendency to hold reading materials at arm's length, blurred vision at normal reading distance, and eye fatigue along with headaches when doing close work. Nearsighted people with presbyopia must take off their glasses to read easily.

Age-related macular degeneration (AMD) is a disease that blurs the sharp, central vision you need to read and drive. The condition affects the macula, the part of the eye that allows you to see fine detail. There are two treatments for AMD: laser surgery and photodynamic therapy.

VISION CORRECTION

"For men in mid-life, LASIK can permanently correct distance vision. Standard LASIK can be used to give some relief from bifocals by making one eye nearsighted and one eye in focus at a distance for what is called monovision. With increasing age, people with monovision have blurring either for reading or for intermediate distance."—Allen Greenbaum, MD

According to Dr. Greenbaum, refractive procedures may be looked at in two ways:

- Laser procedures can be lumped together as one—either using LASIK or PRK/Epi-LASEK techniques—or as two separate procedures
- CK (conductive keratoplasty) and intraocular lens implants

LASIK provides excellent vision, which is realized almost immediately. It can be used to correct nearsightedness, farsightedness, and astigmatism. It may not be performed if the cornea is too thin or in the presence of certain corneal disease. It should not be performed in cases of significant dry eye. PRK can be performed in those cases where the cornea is too thin or the eye is too dry. Both procedures provide excellent vision and may be performed using "custom" wavefront treatments. PRK, however, is associated with more post-operative pain and longer time to visual recovery.

CK uses radio waves to alter the shape of the cornea to provide better reading ability in patients over forty years of age. It is used in patients who do not require glasses for distance. Only one eye is treated in a technique known as monovision (or blended vision).

Intraocular lenses are mostly used in patients who are too nearsighted to have vision correction done by a laser procedure. Lenses may be inserted into the front chamber of the eye without removing the patient's lens. Clear lens exchange may be performed by removing the patient's own lens and then inserting the appropriate power lens into the back chamber of the eye. The indications for these lenses may expand with the advent of multifocal and accommodating implants which will provide distance, intermediate, and near vision correction.

Sun Protection for Your Eyes

If you really want to be comfortable in the glare and protect your eyes from future cataracts, there is more to selecting sunglasses than having a great fashion sense.

If the cells in the lens of the eye are damaged, they are never replaced.

Damage from ultraviolet and (to a lesser degree) infrared rays can build up over a lifetime and gradually create cloudy areas on your lens. It is hard to see through cataracts and they often must be removed surgically. Macular degeneration—another eye condition resulting from damage to the retina—may also be accelerated by too much unfiltered sun blasting onto the retinas.

TIPS FROM DR. ALLEN GREENBAUM ON SAVING YOUR SIGHT

- The goal is to guard against ultraviolet rays. Filter as much of this as you can away from your eyes

- Most sunglasses coated with UV blockers will block the ultraviolet B rays, but the cheaper ones may cheat a little on ultraviolet A rays

- Some contact lenses also block UVB

- Brightness is also an issue. Going from inside to outside involves confronting light thousands of times brighter than that going into the eye the moment before. It is uncomfortable to go into the sun from the shade and to have undimmed light flowing into your eyes

- Clear glass transmits 90 percent of light. As the glasses get darker, less and less light goes through. Lightly tinted lenses let in 75 percent to 80 percent of light. The best glasses are in the 20 percent range. The overall best color to get is gray which absorbs light across the spectrum equally

- Polarized sunglasses are very helpful against reflected light (such as on water, snow, or the road). The light particles called photons travel in a wave form. Polarized sunglasses have a protective layer bonded on them—much like the tinted film put on car windshields—and they admit only vertical waves. Since most reflected waves come in horizontally, those waves are blocked

CHAPTER 5

Enhancing Facial Features

The goal of facial surgery is to enhance the natural structure of the face and create harmony.

CHIN & JAW ENHANCEMENT

Facial height, width, and symmetry are measured by first examining the face from its front and then from the side to determine the facial lateral width or projection of your profile, and contours such as the cheek bones, chin, and nose as well as the eyes, eyebrows, forehead, lips, chin, and neck. This information is then used to determine the best procedure or combination of procedures to achieve the best look for you.

For men whose chin is out of proportion to their nose, or who would prefer a more defined feature, chin and jaw enhancement are options. The facial profile can be balanced by extending the chin in proportion to the nose. Along with chin surgery, some men elect to have the lower jawbone repositioned (reconstructive mandibular sliding surgery) to correct biting and chewing dysfunctions. Sometimes liposuction is used to remove fat and produce a more sharply defined chin and jawline.

CHIN AUGMENTATION

A chin augmentation involves placing a synthetic or biological implant to make the bone structure of the lower face, including the lower jaw, more prominent. Your facial dimensions and natural facial shape are taken into account to determine the placement as well as the size and contour of the chin implants. The result creates a balance, a more defined face. Originally, chin implants were used for reconstruction for birth defects and trauma related incidents. Now, they are used to enhance a man's chin or to create symmetry within the facial structure from a weak chin. With a chin implant, the face is changed into a more aesthetically pleasing and balanced shape.

To be a candidate for a chin augmentation, you must not have any bone disorders, and you must not be or have been on Accutane® for acne for six months or longer because it can cause excessive facial bone growth and increased keloid-like scarring after incisions.

Chin implants are commonly made from solid silicone or other materials. The procedure is commonly performed using twilight anesthesia but when combined with other procedures, general anesthesia is recommended. The chin augmentation procedure takes from one to one and a half hours to perform. Depending upon your facial structure the incisions is placed as inconspicuously as possible. An incision is made inside the lower lip or under the chin. The implant is placed directly on top of the bone and either sutured or screwed into place.

Chin surgery can be approached in several ways. One technique is to make an incision inside the mouth along the groove inside the lower gum to gain access to the chin bone; then a horizontal cut (called an osteotomy) is made through the jawbone with a bone saw or chisel. Next, the lower portion of the separated bone is moved forward to the desired position and wired or screwed into place with titanium plates. The mental nerves are carefully protected. Because the incision is made inside the mouth, there is no visible scarring and the incisions tend to heal much faster when made externally. The risk of infection, however, is higher if an incision is placed within the mouth area. A strict post-operative oral hygiene regimen can decrease this risk.

Another option is to make the incision underneath the chin for a "sliding genioplasty" or chin advancement surgery. This surgery utilizes a bone saw to trim a piece off the bottom of the chin, "slides" it forward, and then fastens it with titanium screws. Metal plates may also be used as well. Although a rarity, bone infection is a risk.

A simple procedure uses an artificial chin implant. After the incision is made, a pocket is created in front of the chin bone and under the muscles and then an appropriately sized chin implant is inserted. The incision is closed with sutures and an external pressure dressing applied. Dissolvable sutures may be used in the surrounding tissues. If no internal sutures are used, tape or a chinstrap is worn longer unless the pocket fits the implant snugly.

There is normally some pain related to a chin implant and pain medication is prescribed. The swelling begins to disappear within the first five to seven days but may be apparent for weeks and the final look may not become evident for a month or two. Numbness may be felt but that usually disappears within one to three months.

The sutures, if any, are removed after three to five days. Many patients return to work after about five days. Regular activities can be resumed after one to two weeks, and exercise after three weeks. We instruct our male patients to avoid scheduling high profile events for at least four weeks after surgery.

The results are immediate, although men tend to think the implant is too small at first glance. After the mind has time to recognize the difference between swelling and augmentation, most are very satisfied with the augmentation results. Silicone chin implants are made to last a lifetime, especially if the implants are of the harder variety and screwed into place, which minimize the risk of shifting.

If the implant moves or if the patient is not happy with the results, additional surgery can be performed to correct or improve the results of a previous chin enhancement procedure.

Common Problems with Chin Implants

- Implant is too large
- Implant is too small
- Asymmetry (uneven)
- Wrong implant type
- Implant displacement
- Implant extrusion
- Infection
- Thickened scars

JAW IMPLANTS

When a chin implant alone is not sufficient to further define the face, a jaw implant can be used in place of or in addition to a chin augmentation. A jaw or mandibular augmentation involves placing an implant or bone graft to make the jawbone structure more prominent. It can balance an otherwise less defined face or further augment an already existing mandibular structure. Because there are quite a few types, sizes, and models available—although not nearly as many as with chin implants—the implant used is most appropriate for the facial shape and desired results. As with a chin implant, the face is measured and the type of implant used is determined based upon the width and symmetry of both the front and side views of the face.

Most jaw augmentations are performed with twilight anesthesia, although general anesthesia can be used. Depending upon the extent of the procedure, the technique used, and the type of implant selected, the procedure takes one to two hours to perform. The incision is made in the predetermined place, the implant is situated directly on top of the bone (or right on top the overlying tissue covering it), and either sutured or screwed into place. The incision is closed with a non-dissolvable type suture. A tape or a head wrapping is worn post-operatively during the day for the recovery period and at night to help it heal properly.

After surgery, the patient has to take it easy and sleep on two pillows to keep the head elevated for seven to fourteen days. the lower face is very swollen for the first three days. Swelling and bruising dissipate over the first few weeks. Some discomfort for several weeks. If the incision is made in the mouth, the diet may be restricted. Fresh fruits and vegetables should be washed, and one should not eat raw fish (sushi), very rare meat, or any other types of foods that may contain high amounts of bacteria. Eating these may increase the risk of infection since the incisions are in the mouth. One may be instructed to rinse with mouthwash several times a day. Keep the hands and tongue away from the incisions or sutures.

MANLY NOSES

If that bump on the nose or if the profile seems to be dwarfing the chin, nasal refinement procedures are on the rise. Once thought of as a rite of passage for teenagers, rhinoplasty has increased in popularity among adult men. A subtle improvement in the shape of the nose can make a huge impact on the overall appearance.

In men, I tend to avoid dramatic changes. Wide, crooked, or protruding nasal bones can be realigned to create a more distinguished look to the nose. If the nose needs to be built up or enlarged in certain areas, I may use grafts of cartilage or synthetic materials. The bones and cartilage are skillfully narrowed, and the skin and soft tissues will redrape themselves over the bony architecture of the new nasal shape. I can correct breathing problems at the same time by removing any internal obstructions (deviated septum or enlarged turbinates). Nasal operations are often combined with a chin implant to improve facial contours and proportions; the projection of the nose is reduced and the chin projection is extended for a more balanced and masculine appearance.

As fashions and beauty standards have evolved over the years, the definition of an attractive female nose has changed as well, but the handsome male nose has remained unchanged since the Renaissance. In male nasal aesthetics, a masculine nose is characterized on profile by a strong upper nose. The desired dorsal line is either straight or has a small bony hump. Dorsal height is considered desirable, as most male patients—even those with mild saddling from birth or as a result of a previous rhinoplasty—request dorsal augmentation. Men often specifically request that a little hump be preserved to maintain a natural looking nose.

Another option is to augment the tip of the nose to include a nasal tip rotation or cartilage graft. To ensure subtly and masculinity, the nasal tip rotation should never give a turned-up appearance to the nose, and a nasolabial angle of at most 90 degrees is preferable. On the other hand, an acute nasolabial angle that creates a droopy nasal tip gives the appearance of an unattractive, sagging nose that can prematurely age a man. The secret is to find a balance between turned up and droopy.

MALE TALE: Stephen is a 34-year old professor of American studies in a small college in upstate New York. When he was a teenager on the hockey team at school, he had an injury and broke his nose badly. It never healed right and left him with a large bump and a twisted tip. "My nose looks like I went two rounds with Tony Soprano," says Stephen, "it really shakes my confidence, especially when meeting a new lady." His mother was a longtime patient of mine and suggested that he come in for a consultation. Stephen had one of the noses that plastic surgeons love to do because we know we can make a big difference in his appearance. When I looked inside his nose, I told Stephen that I was surprised he was able to breathe. His previous injury had narrowed his nasal valves and his septum was severely deviated. Stephen was not convinced he should do it until I showed him a series of photos of another nose I had done that had a similar problem. "Wow, I never realized that it could look that much better," he said. It was about a year later when he finally did have the surgery. One year after that, I got a wedding announcement from Stephen and his new bride, along with a thank you note from his mother who credited me for helping Stephen get his personal life on track. One year later, I got a baby announcement, and another note from Stephen's mother thanking me for giving her a grandchild.

Most men prefer a strong, balanced facial profile that gives the impression of personal confidence. Those who recognize that a weak or receding chin gives a diminutive or passive image often grow a beard or goatee to hide this deficiency. Chin augmentation can be performed simultaneously with a rhinoplasty to bring the face into better alignment. In some cases, one may not recognize the value of a prominent chin and identify the nose as the offending feature, especially because it looks larger in comparison to the receding chin. Chin augmentation actually gives me license to reduce the dorsum less, which is particularly helpful in those with thick skin that might not retract with a greater cartilage or bony removal. Typically, the less the dorsal reduction, the more masculinity is preserved.

CHAPTER 6

Quick Fixes with Fillers & Botulinum Toxin

Non-surgical treatments have become increasingly popular with men due to the lack of downtime and simplicity associated with them.

HOW FILLERS WORK

Soft tissue fillers are injected at different levels of the skin and subcutaneous tissue. They plump up sunken tissue, soften wrinkles and furrows, reduce scars, and fill the hollows of the face. Where each product is placed depends on a variety of factors, including the type of product used and the nature of the correction being sought. It goes without saying that superficial lines require superficial placement of product while deeper folds require deeper placement. Products such as Perlane®, Juvederm®, and Radiesse® are designed to be placed deep into the skin, whereas other dermal fillers such as CosmoDerm® are placed in the superficial layers of the skin. Sculptra® is a new category of filler that is referred to as volumizers. Sculptra® does not directly replace lost volume but rather stimulates the body to produce collagen following a series of injections.

The filler landscape is getting more crowded and there are many more technologies and products that will be available in the near future.

How Long Do They Last?

Fillers differ not only in where they should be injected but also how long they last, their composition, and a host of other factors that should be considered prior to treatment. This ranges from the short term (human collagen) to the permanent (silicone) and includes everything in between. Typical durations are six months for Restylane, to three or four months for Captique® and Hylaform®, and up to several years for Radiesse® and Sculptra®.

What Are the Side Effects?

Injection of soft tissue augmentation products may produce some bruising and swelling. In my experience, the degree depends on the concentration and chemical composition of the product. If you are taking aspirin or anti-inflammatory drugs, or vitamin E, there is a chance that you will have more bruising at the injection sites. Skin type factors in as well; the thinner the skin, the more bruising may be possible.

Injection of any filler is associated with some discomfort and to minimize this, several products contain lidocaine to provide some anesthesia.

I offer my patients pain relief ranging from custom formulated creams to local anesthetic injections that afford a basically pain-free experience. Most men prefer to be comfortable during the treatment.

What Is the Downtime?

The initial downtime following a dermal filler treatment depends upon the amount of material injected, the location of the injection, and the type of material used. Any soft tissue injection may produce asymmetries, swelling, and lumps, although this is rare and usually related to the technique used. Asymmetry is most typically the result of asymmetric swelling, with one side of the face swelling more than the other, which usually corrects itself within a few weeks. Swelling is most common with thicker products and when injecting the lips. Treatment of the swollen areas usually consists of applying ice and taking a non-steroidal anti-inflammatory. Applying ice after a treatment injection will help reduce swelling, bruising, and discomfort. We always recommend that patients avoid having treatments done right before important events or travel plans.

What Fillers Go Where

Every plastic surgeon or dermatologist has his or her favorite fillers. I will select a filler based on my own experience as well as on the patient's goals, financial situation, and experiences. In general, thicker substances are best for deep creases or areas that need long-lasting correction as well as for sculpting cheekbones and augmenting lips. Thinner substances such as Captique®, Hylaform®, CosmoDerm®, and Zyderm® work better for fine lines and superficial wrinkles. They are also a good choice for areas where the skin is thin, such as around the eyelids and lips. Intermediate and thick products such as Restylane®, Perlane®, and Radiesse® work well for deep creases including the marionette lines or nasolabial creases.

The variety of fillers creates an imperative to understand the differences among them in order to decide which ones might be right for you. My preference is to use only safe, effective, and well-established dermal fillers as an alternative as well as an adjunct to surgical results.

HYALURONIC ACIDS

Hyaluronic acid is a natural polysaccharide (sugar molecule) that is an important structural element of the skin, subcutaneous tissue, connective tissue, synovial tissue, and joint fluid. Hyaluronic acid functions in the body to bind water and lubricate joints, and its composition is identical in all living organisms. The chains of sugars that form hyaluronic acids are cross linked together to prevent them from being rapidly degraded. One way that various hyaluronic acids differ is the location and extent of this cross linkage. Hyaluronic acid in its pure form is *highly* bio-compatible and requires no pre-treatment allergy testing.

It is logical to use hyaluronic acids to replace lost volume for a variety of reasons. They are well tolerated, easy to inject, long lasting, and, most importantly, they replace what the body has lost. The various hyaluronic acid products differ in the amount of material they contain as well as their origins. The source of the material may be from animals (e.g., rooster combs in the case of Hylaform® and Hylaform® Plus), or bacterial fermentation (in the case of Restylane® products and Captique®).

The most common areas to treat in men are the nasolabial folds (creases from the nose to mouth), the lips, the oral commissure creases (corners of the mouth), around the lips, and cheek and chin contours.

Since there is no anesthetic supplied in the syringe, my male patients typically require some pain relief, especially in the lip area. Aside from the usual temporary redness or puffiness for the first day or two, we see very few complications from this material.

Restylane®

The FDA approval of Restylane® marked the beginning of a wave of new bioengineered substances for the treatment of lines, depressions, and wrinkles. Restylane®, Perlane®, and Restylane Touch are all the same molecule packaged in a different particle size. To help picture what this means, imagine a block of Jell-O being pushed through a screen. If the screen size is larger, the particles will be big as with Perlane®. If the screen size is smaller, the size of the Jell-O particles will be smaller, as with Restylane®. No matter how you push the gel through the screen, it is the same gel. In general, it is best to use the larger particles to fill deep wrinkles and the smaller ones to fill superficial lines.

My male patients are very satisfied with the results of Restylane®, which lasts six months or longer in most cases. I use Restylane® to treat nasolabial creases (smile lines) and to sculpt cheek bones. By using Restylane® injections along the cheek bone, I can frequently get the entire face to lift up by as much as a millimeter or two. This usually provides dramatic results that last for several months. The effects of Restylane® may be further extended by using Botox® in order to limit muscles that would otherwise cause skin wrinkling. Perlane® is ideal for restoring volume to the cheeks, chin, and jawline. It is used for deep creases including the nasolabial creases and for facial sculpting. It is currently not available in the United States—but FDA approval is soon expected.

Restylane® is the only product approved for use in the United States at the time of this printing, however since Perlane® and Restylane Touch are the exact same molecule, we expect them to be approved soon.

Restylane Sub Q®

The latest addition to the expanding Restylane® family of hyaluronic acid fillers is SubQ®, a revolutionary new injectable treatment for facial sculpting. It can produce the higher cheek bones or a more defined chin and jaw-line.

Restylane SubQ® is based on the same patented hyaluronic acid gel formula used in the other Restylane products but it has much larger gel particles that are three times as thick as Perlane®. SubQ® can also be used for restoring facial volume where cheeks have hollowed from weight loss and the inevitable breakdown of collagen and elastin fibers. The gel is injected deeply under the skin under a local anesthetic in one treatment, and the newly enhanced contours are immediate. At the time of this printing, Restylane SubQ® is available in Europe but not yet approved in the United States.

Hylaform® and Hylaform® Plus

Hylaform® and Hylaform® Plus are hyaluronic acids that are derived from an animal source, i.e. rooster combs. Hylaform® Plus has a larger particle size and is designed for deeper creases. Correction typically lasts four months.

Captique®

Captique® is basically the same as Hylaform® with the major difference that it is manufactured rather than harvested from rooster combs. This allows the product to be produced without any animal proteins that theoretically can cause allergic reactions. It is the same concentration and thickness as Hylaform® and lasts about as long.

Juvederm®

Juvederm® is a homogenous gel that does not contain gel particles. It is manufactured and is not derived from animals. Three versions are presently available, and they are well suited to a broad range of applications. The versions are known as Juvederm® 18, 24, and 30, and they vary in their concentration of hyaluronic acid. Juvederm® is currently undergoing clinical trials in the United States.

COLLAGENS

Collagen is one of the key ingredients in the connective tissue of the skin. Products used for collagen replacement include the original bovine (cow) form of collagen as well as products derived from human skin or cultured from one's own skin. Due to their short longevity, I do not typically recommend these products for my male clients, who prefer to have longer lasting treatments so they do not have to come back as often for treatments.

Bovine Collagen

Bovine collagen was the original soft-tissue augmentation product approved in the United States. There are three types of collagen: Zyderm® I, Zyderm® II and Zyplast®. Since 3 percent of patients may be allergic to bovine (cow) collagen, skin testing is required before treatment. Double skin tests are usually performed about two weeks apart. Therefore, it takes about one month to have the first treatment. Bovine collagen lasts about three or more months on average.

CosmoDerm®/CosmoPlast®

These fillers contain human collagen that has been purified from a human fibroblast cell culture. Like the products derived from cows, they contain 0.3% lidocaine. Unlike Zyderm® and Zyplast®, these products do not require testing and this is their major advantage. CosmoDerm® has the same concentration as Zyderm I, and it is used the exact same way. CosmoPlast® is similar to Zyplast® and is used in the same way. Typically, CosmoDerm® and CosmoPlast® last up to four months.

Using One's Own Cells

Isolagen

Isolagen is made with cultured autologous fibroblasts to produce viable connective tissue cells, collagen, and other products needed for dermal support. The process begins with a small skin sample typically taken from behind the ear. The specimen is sent to the lab where it is grown and then sent back to the physician's office to be injected into the skin. This product has great potential for long-term correction of soft tissue defects. Clinical trials are underway that may lead to FDA approval in 2007.

VOLUMIZERS

A new category of fillers known as volume enhancers are great for replacing volume in the nasolabial creases and cheeks. They hold promise for treating aging hands as well.

SCULPTRA®

Sculptra® works by stimulating the body to produce collagen to replace what has been lost. Sculptra® is composed of polylactic acid (the same material used for absorbable sutures). Sculptra® is a polymerized lactic acid (PLA) similar to the material used for absorbable sutures for decades. This product was approved for use in HIV patients in the United States in August 2004, although it has been available in Europe for many years. The powdered material is reconstituted into a suspension, which is injected just below the deep dermis. It is used off-label to treat deep facial hollows and creases, although approval for cosmetic uses in the United States is expected soon.

Sculptra® is biocompatible (the body does not see it as foreign), biodegradable, and immunologically inert. It requires a series of three injections spaced between four and six weeks apart. Once Sculptra® is injected, the body is stimulated to produce its own collagen and thereby fill in depressed creases of the face. Long-term correction with Sculptra® may last eighteen to twenty-four months.

AUTOLOGOUS FAT TRANSFER

Fat transfers can be a valuable technique for major volume restoration, as in cheeks, lips, and hollows. This requires a minor procedure to obtain one's own fat. The fat is then cleaned and carefully re-injected into areas of the face that need more fullness. Reinjected fat lasts longer in larger areas of non-movement, so it is very successful for the correction of sunken cheeks and lipoatrophy. Fat transfer can also correct aging of the hands.

Patients are up and around immediately following fat injections. There may be some swelling and bruising. Results may last six months to several years, and usually, multiple treatment sessions are needed.

SEMI-PERMANENT AND PERMANENT FILLERS

Fillers engineered to last for years or even decades are now being used with the goal of reducing the number of patient visits required to obtain soft tissue augmentation. Long-term consequences including granulomas, lumps, and infections may arise with some of these products. I am cautious about using these products because of their potential for permanence. If they migrate, the only way to remove them is through surgery.

Radiesse®

Radiesse® is composed of calcium hydroxyl apatite (CAHA) made from calcium and phosphate. This product has been used for multiple indications including craniofacial surgery (repair of the bones of the face and head) and cheek and chin implants. CAHA is the naturally occurring matrix found in bones, and it is biocompatible. The particles are in a gel carrier made up of cellulose, glycerin, and purified water. The results feel soft, and natural correction can be achieved in one treatment. I use Radiesse® for men in the nasolabial folds (nose-to-mouth lines), oral commissures (marionette lines), chin creases and to smooth out the contours of the jaw line. I have used it for very deep frown lines with impressive results in men. Radiesse® lasts approximately one year. It can also be used to strengthen the chin and cheekbones.

Artefill®

ArteFill® consists of polymethylmethacrylate microspheres (PMMA), tiny beads of plexiglass suspended in bovine collagen. The collagen is degraded by the body within three months, and the PMMA microspheres remain. ArteFill® is implanted into the deep dermis with a needle and then massaged and molded to the contour desired. It is used for acne scars, nasolabial folds, and depressions such as sunken cheeks. At the present time, FDA is expected very soon.

Injectable Liquid Silicone

Liquid silicones with varying degrees of purity have been used to treat wrinkles and scars for decades. The attraction of the product is that it is permanent. Newer methods of injection, referred to as the micro droplet technique, have the advantage of causing fewer lumps than prior techniques. Although permanent correction of nasolabial creases sounds appealing, there are risks inherent with permanent fillers. The prospect of having to excise the silicone if it migrates, becomes infected, or you do not like the way it looks is daunting. Adatosil-5000 and Silikon-1000 are approved for use as ophthalmic devices. Therefore, applying it for cosmetic purposes is considered off-label usage.

LONG-TERM RESULTS

The key to successful long-term results with dermal fillers is an understanding of which product is best for an individual patient's goals, skin and temperament. For the most part, I have found that men do best with thicker, more viscous fillers since their skin tends to be thicker with deeper creases and folds, and fewer superficial wrinkles. My filler of choice for men is Restylane®, and I also get excellent results using Radiesse® in men.

CHAPTER 7

Sculpting the Torso

"Middle age is when your age starts to show around your middle." —Bob Hope

Body type is determined largely by genetics, over which we have no control. Every man is born with one of three basic body types: ectomorph, mesomorph, and endomorph.

MALE BODY TYPES

- Ectomorph is the type that fashion magazines would have us aspire to: tall with long thin limbs and little body fat. Basketball players are the ectomorph body type

- Mesomorph body types are characterized by an athletic, strong, and compact body. Tennis players tend to fall into the mesomorph category

- Endomorphs are round and gain weight easily

The body type of birth with is the body type that you will have for life. It is a physical characteristics, just like eye color.

Human growth hormone (hGH) is produced by the pituitary gland and is important to the growth process from birth through adolescence. A deficiency of hGH increases the volume of fat and abdominal obesity that men store and reduces muscle mass and strength. A drop in the natural production of hGH is a direct pathway to producing flab around the middle, and natural production decreases inexplicably starting in the early twenties.

THE CHEST WALL

Affecting almost 40 percent of men, gynecomastia is the most common breast problem in men, especially during adolescence. It is defined as the unilateral or bilateral enlargement of the male breast. The male breast appears fuller and rounded compared with the ideal flattened and rectangular male breast contour. Typically, gynecomastia is caused by a combination of dense breast tissue behind the nipple and fatty tissue over the pectoralis major muscle. The fullness of the male breast is detected by firmness just below the nipple, and extends around the side to the edge of the pectoralis muscle and into the armpits.

In pseudogynecomastia, breast enlargement is principally the result of excess fat accumulation. True gynecomastia is a proliferation of the glandular breast tissue with or without increased fat accumulation. Most often, men do not have any underlying medical or hormonal problems and the patient's concern is primarily the aesthetic appearance. They want a flatter, more defined breast and chest shape as well as flatter and smaller nipples and areola (the pigmented area of the nipple).

UNDERLYING CAUSES FOR THE DEVELOPMENT OF GYNECOMASTIA

- Drug-Induced
- Antiretroviral therapy
- Androgenic steroids
- Spironolactone
- Cimetidine
- Alkylating agents
- Oral contraceptives
- Digitalis
- Marijuana, heroin
- Estrogens
- Estrogen-testosterone imbalance
- Increased estrogen secretion states
- Increased peripheral conversion to estrogen
- Hermaphroditism
- Klinefelter's syndrome
- Congenital adrenal hyperplasia
- Adrenal disease
- Liver disease
- Thyrotoxicosis
- Hormone-producing neoplasms
- Neoplasm
- Testicular tumors
- Reduced testosterone production or activation

DR. JACOBS' CLASSIFICATION OF GYNECOMASTIA

I. a) Thickened tissues directly below the areola

   b) Thickened tissue extending beyond the areolar edge

II. Moderate breast enlargement; no skin redundancy; volume of excess tissue approximately the size of a squashed baseball

III. Moderate breast enlargement; minor skin redundancy; volume of excess tissue approximately the size of a squashed softball

IV. Gross breast enlargement, severe skin redundancy; volume of excess tissue approximately the size of a squashed dodgeball

NOTE: A "B" category for II—IV indicates droop of the nipples below the breast fold.

Men may be embarrassed and feel extremely self-conscious about their feminized appearing chest. When dealing with adolescents, the psychological burden is often very apparent and can lead to social isolation and low self-esteem. Concerned parents sometimes report that their sons withdraw from peers to avoid the gym or visits to the pool or beach. The slang term "man-boobs" has become part of the vernacular to describe a man with a fatty, protruding chest that resembles female breasts.

Most of the men I see fall into Class II and III in the Classification Chart above. I always perform the physical exam in a warm room so the nipple is relaxed. A contracted nipple may mask mild to moderate gynecomastia.

In order to determine the appropriate treatment, I have to examine the breast thoroughly to determine the prominent tissue types and to evaluate the size of the breast enlargement. If the medical history or physical exam imply a possible underlying medical problem, I may suggest further diagnostic testing. Correcting gynecomastia requires an individually tailored approach for each patient's needs.

In general, adolescents with visible breast enlargement most commonly have a glandular type or combination of glandular-fatty type detected. Around middle age, men tend to accumulate more fatty tissue, although sometimes a combination of glandular and fatty tissue causes the breast enlargement.

What Can Be Done?

There are multiple surgical approaches for the treatment of gynecomastia. Surgery to reduce the size of the male breast can be done in an out patient surgical facility; local or general anesthesia is used. Aggressive liposuction alone may be sufficient in some cases. I use traditional tumescent liposuction with specialized cannulae that I have designed for this procedure. I have found that the use of ultrasonic assisted liposuction (UAL) only helps to melt fat and has no effect on breast tissue. There is a fallacy that UAL makes gynecomastia surgery easier, but it can actually be less effective. UAL alone may sometimes lead to disappointing results since it helps melt fat but not breast tissue.

In cases where liposuction alone is not effective, minimal incision surgery is used to remove the firm breast tissue through an incision that is hidden at the edge of the areola. The areolar approach provides a more cosmetically pleasing result since the scar does not extend into the surrounding skin. Since it is important that the incision does not extend into the neighboring tissue, the length of the incision is limited, and the surgery is more difficult.

Given the psychological ramifications of gynecomastia, the aesthetic outcome is one of the key end points, so overt scarring and landmark deformities should be avoided. A combination approach, consisting of tumescent liposuction followed by sharp excision of the breast nugget through an incision in the nipple, is very common. The incision allows for direct removal of firm breast tissue, and the liposuction is used to feather and taper the contours. This approach produces aesthetically pleasing results for men with glandular and mixed gynecomastia. In cases with more advanced gynecomastia, patients may benefit considerably from liposuction alone because there is significant skin reduction that results from skin contraction after liposuction. Skin excisions are rarely needed in most patients. The presented combination technique is a safe and aesthetically satisfying approach for the treatment of gynecomastia that often produces a long lasting outcome.

GETTING BACK TO WORK

After surgery, a light compression garment is worn for several weeks as a dressing. Patients can resume normal activities within days and even shower two days after surgery. Peaking at two to three days, swelling is mild to moderate and disappears rapidly over the next three weeks. Minimal or no bruising is common. Dissolving sutures are placed under the skin so there are no sutures to remove. After swelling disappears, expect a permanent balanced and proportioned contour. There will be some firmness in all the treated areas. Although not visible, this firmness will take several more months to resolve.

MALE TALE: Roger, age 38, is a successful real-estate broker who is thrilled to be the father a 7-year-old girl named Jennifer, who is an avid swimmer. In fact, Jennifer's coach expected her to qualify for her school's swim team in a few years. Due to the bulky shape of his chest, Roger had not been near a pool himself since college. Although not terribly overweight, Roger had a stocky, muscular build and well-developed biceps. Unfortunately, he also had excess fatty deposits on his chest wall which caused him to cover up at the gym, beach, and poolside. As swimming was becoming a more important part of Jennifer's life, he started to feel pressure to throw on a pair of Speedos and lose the baggy tee shirt he always wore in order to spend more time with her. After seeing a segment about Dr. Jacob's treatment of gynecomastia on 20/20, Roger was surprised to realize that he was not alone. He had lived most of his life with the idea that his chest did not look like every other guy's, when in fact, there were actually many men just like him. Roger came to my office for a consultation, and he was even embarrassed to take his shirt off in the exam room. "I expected Dr. Jacobs to say it was the worst case he had ever seen, but instead, he made me feel relaxed about the whole thing," says Roger." My daughter was my real motivation. I didn't want to watch her grow up making excuses for why I couldn't go swimming with her. "Roger scheduled his surgery right after Jennifer was going away to swimming camp. When visiting day came, he surprised her by diving into the Olympic sized pool. "The big smile on her face was something I'll never forget," he says.

MALE BREAST CANCER

Most people do not realize that men have breast tissue and that they can develop breast cancer.

In fact, 1 percent of all breast cancers occur in men. About 1,500 cases of breast cancer and 400 breast cancer deaths occur in men each year in the United States.

Until puberty, young boys and girls have a small amount of breast tissue consisting of a few ducts (tubular passages) located under the nipple and areola (pigmented skin around the nipple). At puberty, a girl's ovaries produce female hormones, causing breast tissue to grow, while male hormones produced by the testes prevent further growth of breast tissue. Like all cells of the body, a man's breast duct cells can undergo cancerous changes. Because women have many more breast cells than men do—and perhaps because their breast cells are constantly exposed to the growth-promoting effects of female hormones—breast cancer is much more common in women. Men with a history of testicular or breast disease, a family history of breast cancer in women, or Jewish ancestry have a higher-than-average risk for developing breast cancer. Men with a genetic condition called Klinefelter syndrome have a much higher risk for breast cancer. The presence of gynecomastia, however, does not increase the risk of breast cancer.

PEC IMPLANTS

Male chest enhancement is growing in popularity as more men are choosing to enhance their physiques, body symmetry, and self-image with pectoral implants. Pectoral implants offer a more prominent and muscular appearing chest as well as an opportunity to correct unevenness from one side to the other. This procedure can enhance a patient with an already shapely physique but who just cannot achieve the chest bulk he desires through weight lifting. Or, pectoral implants may be used to simulate the effects of spending hours at the gym. It can be combined with reducing the size of the nipples and areolae, or other plastic surgery procedures.

Who Is the Ideal Candidate?

An ideal candidate for pectoral implants is a man who is dissatisfied with his underdeveloped chest and who is free of any complicating, pre-existing medical conditions including heart disease, high blood pressure, diabetes, and skin or connective tissue disorders. Pec implants, as they are called, involve inserting a soft, high grade, solid silicone implant into a space created under the pectoral muscles. To the touch, it has the feeling and consistency of a flexed muscle. Unlike female breast augmentation, after this procedure is properly completed and healed, there is no reason to require additional surgery in the future. Frequently liposuction of the love handles, abdomen, waist, and back, or any combination is performed to further enhance the overall shape and contour of the torso.

These implants are made of soft silicone block so that they cannot leak or spread since there is no gel or fluid. They come in different shapes and sizes to accommodate any anatomic features and the cosmetic look the patient desire. A consultation and physical examination is needed to help determine the most appropriate size and shape. Generally, scars are easily hidden in the armpit area within the hair bearing skin. The initial consultation is extremely important to review the patient's medical history, goals, and expectations, as well as to build mutual trust and rapport. A complete evaluation and physical examination is performed for each individual patient to insure that expectations can be met, as well as to determine the best choice of procedures. The size and shape of the implants to be used are determined next. I review the surgical plan as well as the incisions or scar placement with the patient. Although every effort is made to accomplish the desired set of goals, no guarantees as to the exact size, projection, and contour of the male chest can be made by any surgeon.

How Is the Surgery Performed?

This procedure is usually performed on an out patient basis, under general anesthesia or local anesthesia with intravenous sedation. The surgery generally takes approximately one and one half hours. The surgical plan, including implant placement and incision lines, is outlined before surgery. When asleep, local nerve blocks combined with medication that shrinks blood vessels and capillaries to reduce bleeding are instilled. An incision high in the armpit, about two inches long, is used to create a space between the two chest wall muscles—the pectoralis major and the pectoralis minor. The implant is placed between these two muscles. It is well camouflaged and safe in this position. A "pocket" or space is created under each pectoral muscle of the chest corresponding to the planned outline on the skin, which was marked prior to surgery. The solid silicone pectoral implants are then inserted. The incision is closed with sutures below the level of the skin to avoid cross-hatching and suture marks. Liposuction, or any other procedures, are performed next. At the conclusion of surgery a light dressing and elastic compression garment is applied over the surgical area. These are easily concealed and are worn for about three to four weeks or less. The results are immediately visible.

Getting Back to Work

Following the surgery, patients generally report mild to moderate pain which is easily controlled with medication and rapidly subsides after two days. Varying degrees of swelling and generally mild bruising peak at two to three days and then subside over several weeks. Gentle arm raising maneuvers begin immediately after surgery. You can shower and wash in two days. The elastic compression garment or bandage is generally worn for one to two weeks following surgery. Routine activities may be resumed after two weeks, and some lower body exercise can be resumed in two to three weeks. Full workouts are permissible somewhere between four to six weeks. Recovery and healing will vary from patient to patient. Complete healing often takes several months before the final results of surgery are apparent. Expect a normal result that does not look artificial or unusual even when flexing or working the muscles, and that does not change or sag over time.

What Are the Possible Risks?

Possible complications include: anesthesia risks, bleeding, infection, fluid accumulation under the skin (seroma) which may need to be drained, nerve damage, poor wound healing, and unsatisfactory scars. Asymmetry, displacement, hardening of the scar tissue around the implant, and the need for revisional surgery or even removal of the implants are also possible. Venodyne calf compression devices are often used for pectoral implant surgery (as well as many other surgeries). Venodynes are pressure cuffs that fit over each lower leg from the ankle to the knee circulating every one to two minutes to reduce the pooling of blood in the lower extremities and further reduce the possibility of blood clots or emboli. Smokers must stop smoking well in advance of surgery. Smoking seriously decreases blood circulation in the skin, which increases the risk of complications and poor healing.

BODY SCULPTING VIA LIPOSUCTION

Liposuction can remove love-handles that even exercise addicts cannot shed on their own.

There are a fixed number of adult fat cells distributed in a genetically predetermined fashion throughout the body. As a man gains weight, these cells expand. As he loses weight, the fat cells contract in size, but the number and distribution remain essentially unchanged. Dieting reduces a man's weight and overall size and may show improvement in specific areas. Liposuction, on the other hand, reduces the total number of fat cells and therefore, affects shape and contour so future weight gain or loss will not be noticed as much in the areas that were treated. It is a safe and effective way to remove bulges to produce an improved shape and contour.

Most areas of the body can be suctioned, from the face down to the ankles. Stubborn fat deposits that do not respond to exercise and diet regimens are ideal targets for liposuction. Men tend to accumulate fat deposits around the midsection—typically the abdomen, waist, and chest. These areas are frequently combined in one stage to maximize the potential for the skin to shrink after the fat is removed. However, the typical "beer belly," with fat located within the abdominal cavity, cannot be suctioned at all.

It is also excellent for removing fatty breast tissue and giving men back the abs they had in college. Liposuction can remove stubborn localized fat deposits that working out tirelessly will not budge. Results from liposuction are best if men continue regular workouts at the gym after the procedure. Men often have more resilient skin than women, so it tends to contract better following the procedure, which allows for greater volume removal.

POWER ASSISTED LIPOPLASTY

There has been much discussion about power assisted lipoplasty, or PAL. In my view, it is not any more precise than more traditional methods; it simply makes the surgery less tiresome for the surgeon. I have found that the vibration of the motor held in the surgeon's hand can dull the feeling in his fingertips. In addition, the cannula can loosen periodically at its attachment to the motor, necessitating an unnecessary pause of the surgery while the cannula is tightened.

LipoSelection™ by VASER

This technique utilizes advanced ultrasound technology to create a more precise and kinder way of separating fatty tissue. Fat pockets are quickly dissolved and then removed from the abdomen, upper arms, hips, saddlebags, necks, and other areas. Due to its tissue selectivity process, this technology minimizes the possibility of uneven contouring, ripples, lumps, and bumps. Recovery is fast, minimizing pain and bruising and maximizing smooth skin retraction. Most people are able to return to normal activities after a long weekend.

Ultimately, the most important consideration when it comes to getting a great result from liposuction is the skill and aesthetic eye of the surgeon, rather than the instrumentation he or she uses. To have liposuction, one must consider lifestyle, aerobic shape, body/weight fluctuations, and overall health.

Men who are very overweight may have to undergo these procedures in stages. If a patient exceeds his ideal weight by thirty pounds or more, I may advise him to lose weight before having surgery.

RESHAPING THE ABDOMEN & FLANKS

There is a wide variation in the procedures patients can receive, from a clear-cut panniculectomy (removing an apron of skin and fat) to a full abdominoplasty, where I transpose the umbilicus and tighten the muscles of the abdominal wall. There is also variation in the timing of such operations. Some opt for a panniculectomy at the onset, only to be followed by an abdominoplasty later, while others want extensive surgery all at once. The post-bariatric patient does not require a simple 'tummy tuck' in the sense of the cosmetic abdominoplasty surgeries we often perform. The panniculectomy patient has a different set of problems than a tummy tuck patient does.

A panniculectomy has risks that include wound-healing problems and seromas. Of the multitude of plastic surgery procedures available to post-bariatric patients, the abdominal area has received the most attention. The abdominal area presents its own challenges because each post-bariatric case is so different from the next. It really depends on how much weight the patient loses as well as his particular desire. One procedure may require lengthy in-patient surgery while another may be recommended for office-based surgery.

BUTTOCK AUGMENTATION

This is a procedure often done in men who desire a more youthful appearance of the buttock region. This may involve enlargement, reduction, or a lift. Sagging, flabby buttocks related to aging, weight loss, or produced by too much liposuction, can also be improved.

To enlarge the buttocks, the most common procedure is fat grafting, which works extremely well in this area and produces a higher, rounder buttocks. It also lifts sagging buttocks to some degree. Fat is injected into the gluteus muscle and into the fat spaces. Silicone buttock implants can also be placed beneath the muscle through a four-inch incision. Dressings and a light compression garment are worn for several weeks. Expect minimal pain that is mostly gone by the second or third day and is easily controlled by medications. Peaking at two to three days, swelling is mild to moderate and then disappears rapidly over the next three weeks. There is usually minimal bruising. Some grogginess will persist for several days. One can shower on the second day after surgery and may resume most normal activities within the first week, and strenuous activities within three weeks post-surgery.

BUTTOCK REDUCTION

Reducing the buttocks almost always involves liposuction only. This must be done thoroughly, but not overdone to avoid sagging and to achieve a balanced, proportioned buttock. Good skin tone and elasticity are essential in this area. Dressings and a light compression garment are used for several weeks, but there are no stitches to remove. Recovery is very rapid and mostly comfortable, with minimal pain that is mostly gone by the second or third day and is easily controlled by medications. Peaking at two to three days, swelling is mild to moderate and then disappears rapidly over the next three weeks. One can shower on the second day after surgery and can resume many activities within the first week, and most by at least three weeks post-surgery. Expect to be out of work for three to seven days.

WEIGHT LOSS SURGERY

Bariatric or weight loss surgery, performed by specially trained general surgeons, is not really a cosmetic procedure. It works by reducing the size of the stomach and/or digestive tract to limit the intake of calories, thereby resulting in massive weight loss over the course of several months. Obesity is measured by body mass index (BMI). Your BMI is calculated by dividing the weight in kilograms by the height in meters squared. A BMI between 27 and 30 indicates mild obesity, while a BMI of 30 or above indicates more severe obesity with possible health risks. Morbid obesity is indicated by a BMI of 40 or above. Morbid obesity can lead to many life-threatening conditions including: hypertension, heart disease, diabetes, and arthritis. Candidates for gastrointestinal surgery include those with a BMI above 40—approximately 100 pounds overweight for men and 80 pounds for women. In some cases, people with a BMI between 35 and 40 who suffer from type II diabetes or life-threatening cardiopulmonary problems such as severe sleep apnea or obesity-related heart disease may also be candidates for weight-loss surgery. Research has indicated that a 40-inch waist in men indicates an increased risk for heart disease.

Following significant weight loss achieved by gastric bypass or gastric banding, patients typically have significant areas of skin excess. This commonly includes excess skin of the neck, abdomen, breasts, arms, and thighs. Plastic surgeons address these problems with many potential options, including: face and neck lift, abdominoplasty or tummy tuck, breast lifts, gynecomastia reduction, upper arm lift, thigh lifts, and lower body lifts. These patients may also be candidates for other procedures including liposuction and facelifts.

Although the popularity of bariatric surgery has not yet reached its peak, the number of post-bariatric patients seeking plastic surgery-related relief from its effects has grown exponentially. One of the most common complaints with men who have lost a significant amount of weight is that they weigh less and look slimmer overall, but because of skin stretching from weight gain and shrinking from weight loss, unattractive extra skin folds often result. Many times the problem is too severe to be improved sufficiently by traditional methods such as liposuction; instead, a more aggressive procedure is needed to remove redundant skin and produce a pleasing aesthetic look. After significant weight loss, a body lift is usually the only way to get rid of excess skin.

Traditional body-lifting techniques often do not work as well on massive weight-loss patients. Their skin quality and elasticity is different, so when a doctor tightens the skin in a certain area, it may loosen over time. There may be areas that require augmentation in combination with surgical excision. When air is let out of a balloon, it flattens rapidly. However, many men who lose significant amounts of weight—whether by dieting and exercising or through a form of obesity surgery—do not flatten that easily. Surgery is needed to reshape and recontour overly stretched skin, and often more than one surgery is necessary to tackle all the problem areas.

A young man who has a little bit of looseness in the skin may be adequately treated by liposuction. An ideal candidate is a man who can lift up the skin on his thigh and see a significant improvement in the shape and contour. It is also good for a man at a stable weight, for whom the lifting procedure will show clear benefits. It is not a quick fix procedure for an obese man. Whereas liposuction produces a significant drop in clothing size, a body lift often does not because the patient is usually at his final size and just looking to tighten skin.

Body lift surgery produces extensive scarring, but the incisions are usually made in places that can be easily covered by underwear. Since recovery time is often slow, it could take a month or longer before returning to work. Although it depends on many factors including height and age, the best candidates tend to be 190-pound males who have lost a considerable amount of weight. One usually has to wait at least a year or more to have the surgery following a gastric-bypass procedure. Despite the increasing popularity of body lift surgery, it is not appropriate for every man. The patient needs to fully understand what is involved with this kind of surgery before deciding if it is right.

How Is the Surgery Performed?

The body lift procedure entails removing redundant skin and fat from the underlying muscle. The excess skin and fat removal procedure is performed on several areas. First, there is the tummy tuck or abdominoplasty. Then, the inner thigh lift extends from the inner thigh all the way down to the front of the knee. Finally, the lateral thigh and buttock lift is performed. These are usually performed in addition to liposuction. With the body lift procedure, a large portion of the excess skin is removed and then the hanging skin is elevated and tacked much higher. As a result, the wrinkles are removed and the skin is tightened. The body lift does not merely lift and tighten; the excess fat is undermined, lifted off the muscle, and further lifted and elevated. Stitches are placed in several layers of the fibers underneath the skin in the fat or the superficial fascial system (SFS) from below, and attached to the SFS above. This acts as a scaffolding or foundation beneath the skin that holds the fat and skin to the body. When this occurs, the tissues stay in position. The good news is that the incisions are completely hidden in all natural skin creases.

The concept behind the body lift is to first use liposuction to contour the underlying fat, smooth it out, and then lift the looseness around it. If having the entire body lift done, the patient will need to wear a body girdle post-operatively for about two weeks. Lateral thigh and buttock lifts hurt much less than an abdominoplasty because the muscle is not being tightened. The abdominoplasty hurts mostly because the underlying muscle has been tightened. The inner thigh lift hurts quite a bit because the incisions are located where a patient sits. Permanent sutures are placed underneath the skin. With a body lift, the scars tended to be wider than with an abdominoplasty. With permanent sutures in the skin, the scar does not spread—a key component to a good aesthetic result.

There are challenges inherent in the complexity of the surgeries. Most post-bariatric patients undergo plastic surgery after having made a very solid commitment to their health. Although people who have lost a significant amount of body mass may be healthier, there is still a certain amount of risk associated with any body-contouring surgery. Effective surgical treatment requires careful pre-operative, intra-operative and post-operative care. There are no guarantees for any method, including surgery, to produce and maintain weight loss. Success is possible only with hard work and a firm commitment to lifestyle changes.

INNOVATIONS IN NON-SURGICAL LIPOSUCTION

For the past decade, liposuction or lipoplasty has been the most popular surgical procedure worldwide. The concept behind a selection of new devices is to employ ultrasound to treat localized fat deposits without making an incision. These devices (LipoSonix™, UltraShape™) appear to be safe, but further research is needed to determine if the procedure could effect cells other than fat cells. Early results indicate that this technology will be best used for recontouring bulges rather than large volume fat removal.

The injection of phosphatidylcholine (i.e.: mesotherapy) known by the trade name of Lipostabil® or LipoDissolve®, has also been used to dissolve fat in place of surgical intervention. However, physicians have concerns about whether the appropriate amount of fat—neither too little nor too much—is dissolved through these injections, and what the short-term and long-term side effects may be. Claims as to the safety and efficacy of this product have so far not been substantiated by scientific clinical trials in the United States.

AGING AND WEIGHT GAIN

As one ages, the body becomes less muscular and body fat increases. In men, this extra fat is often deposited in the abdominal area. Gaining extra weight accentuates this and results in the spare tire of middle age.

This decrease in muscle mass and increase in fat is the result of several interacting factors. Muscle-building (anabolic) hormones tend to decline with age while muscle-wasting (catabolic) hormones stay constant or increase slightly. These hormonal changes along with diet, exercise, and genetic predisposition cause changes in body composition.

Extra weight around the abdomen or upper body is unhealthy. The distribution of body fat in these areas is associated with an increased risk of heart disease.

An extreme form of changing body composition occurs in Cushing's disease. With this disease, the body is exposed to chronic, very high levels of the catabolic hormone cortisol. Excess fat is deposited in the abdomen, neck, and face while the muscles of your arms and legs waste. Easy bruising, stretch marks, swelling, and an increased risk of diabetes and high blood pressure are associated with this syndrome.

Other conditions—such as liver disease, bowel disorders, and abdominal tumors—can be associated with abdominal enlargement and should not be confused with normal weight gain. If one gains weight around the middle and experiences such signs and symptoms as pain, change in bowel habits, nausea or vomiting, jaundice, leg swelling, urinary problems, or fatigue, see a doctor.

CHAPTER 8

New Skin, New Man

The skin aging process is the same for men and women, but for men it occurs later and is more marked. In a man's skin, the dermis is thicker and richer in collagen, and the epidermis is often more oily.

MEN'S SKIN VS. WOMEN'S SKIN

A man's skin is approximately 20 percent thicker than a woman's, and is typically firmer because it is richer in collagen and elastin. In general, male skin is oilier, with larger pores, a richer blood supply, and an increased tendency to sweat. Men are less prone to wrinkling than women and may require deep cleansing daily. However, because of more active sebaceous glands, men's skin tends to be much oilier. It is also more prone to dehydration because of daily or regular shaving.

A man's skin tends to be more resistant than a woman's skin to the effects of the sun and other environmental factors. Around the age of forty to fifty years, the dermis layer of a man's skin thins, and the level of collagen decreases naturally yet dramatically, causing wrinkles to appear. Just as for women, men can prevent and correct the signs of aging with appropriate skincare. In men, there is a gradual thinning of the skin with increasing age of approximately 1 percent per year.

As men age, wrinkles begin to develop and the skin loses firmness and elasticity. Expression lines form on the face, and patches of discoloration and areas of dilated blood vessels appear. On exposed areas of aged skin, the skin patterns are often markedly changed. Older men may find that deep furrows develop in their skin. Others suffer from the so-called "turkey neck." Smoking has a direct and adverse effect on the skin.

SKIN AGING FACTORS

- Blood circulation slows down
- Metabolism slows down
- Chemical changes take place in the tissues
- Sebaceous glands diminish in size and number
- Collagen production breaks down

A man's skin is his first defense against the effects of the sun, climate, and other environmental factors such as air pollution. The skin fulfils essential functions: body-temperature regulation, elimination of perspiration and toxins, and more. A man's skin needs to be protected effectively and daily.

Good Cleansing

Most men do not want to be bothered with too many skincare products. However, starting with a regimen of basics—cleansing, protection, and moisturizing after shaving—is an effective skincare routine. To a man who simply washes his face with soap and water, this may seem like a complicated regimen. However, the benefits of these few simple steps are abundant.

Daily face washing will keep pores unclogged, which in turn can prevent a variety of skin conditions, from pimples to ingrown hairs. Not only are these painful and unattractive, but they can also leave discolored marks on the skin's surface.

Shaving & Your Skin

Daily shaving can dry out a man's skin. To combat this, look for shaving foams that are specifically designed to treat your skin type, whether it is sensitive skin, dry skin, or skin prone to imperfections. Sensitive skin may be characterized by redness, a burning sensation, and a tendency to experience razor burn. Dry skin may feel tight and lacking in elasticity. Skin prone to imperfections may be characterized by pimples, razor bumps, and ingrown hairs.

After shaving, skin should be soothed with a moisturizer or an aftershave balm. Men's skin should also be protected from the sun for optimum health. Look for a moisturizer with an SPF 15 for daily wear. For sun protection, an SPF 15 or higher broad spectrum sunscreen is recommended for the best protection.

The Right Regimen

Good skincare depends on using products specifically designed to treat your skin type and using them daily to reap the benefits of the products.

Although the skin is a man's first defense, it is the last in line to receive nutrients carried by the blood. It therefore receives vitamins and minerals in small quantities. For the skin to play its role as a vital organ effectively, dermatologists recommend using a daily hydrating moisturizer and a well-balanced supply of targeted vitamins and minerals specially adapted to meet the needs of a man's skin.

SKIN TIPS

- Stick to a basic skincare regimen twice a day, just as women do.

- Men have a built-in advantage in the aging process—their skin is thicker and oilier than women's skin

- Before shaving, take a warm shower or steam the face with a warm cloth to open up the pores. If the water is not warm enough, microwave a damp cloth for about one minute, then test the temperature on the wrist to avoid burning the face

- Never shave with plain water. Apply a protective shaving gel or cream to the face before shaving. In a pinch, lather with soap

- A swivel-head razor is better than a disposable one to decrease nicks. Replace the blade often; a dull blade does not provide a close shave and can be irritating to the skin

- Splashing the face with cold water after shaving closes the pores, but avoid using alcohol-based after-shaves that can burn and dry out skin

ACNE REMEDIES

"There are a number of skin conditions that resemble acne such as eczema, perioral dermatitis, and folliculitis. While they may not involve all of the factors that cause real acne, they do have one thing in common—inflammation. Inflammatory acne starts when the combination of excess skin cells and oil causes pore-aggravating bacteria to develop which leads to pimples, redness, and overall irritation." —Dr. Howard Murad, Los Angeles Dermatologist

Acne is perhaps the fastest growing segment in the skincare realm today, second only to anti-wrinkle products and treatments. Hyperpigmentation can be problematic in darker or bronze skin types. The other principal area of concern is skin sensitivities, such as allergic, reactive, or easily irritated skin.

Types of Acne

Most men see a pimple, and think acne. It is a common mistake to think acne when it could be another skin condition entirely. For example, dermatitis can show up on the lower face and chin in the form of red, inflamed blisters. Blackheads are flat, darkened spots that result from pores becoming plugged with oil, or sebum, and dead skin cells. The dark center of a blackhead is a mixture of dried oil and skin cells that have been shed in the openings of the hair follicles. Blackheads commonly appear on the face, especially around the T-zone, on the bridge of the nose, back, chest, shoulders, and upper arms.

The best treatments for blackheads are aimed at addressing the cause: the processes of oil production and skin cell turnover. Treatment removes skin debris (so it cannot clog the pores), dries the skin, and slows mounting oil production that can become full-blown acne. The goal of acne therapy is to eliminate existing lesions and prevent new ones from forming.

Blackheads—'open comedos' which are formed when dead skin cells and sebum are tightly packed inside a follicle whose walls have broken. If the plug enlarges and pops out of the duct, it is called a blackhead. The skin cells and oil give it a dirty appearance that simply will not wash away.

Whiteheads—'closed comedos' where the plug stays below the surface of the skin so that the follicle wall does not break. Whiteheads are formed on or under the skin.

Papules—red, raised bumps or inflamed lesions that occur when the oily material inside the follicle ruptures into the surrounding skin.

Pustules—similar to papules but slightly more inflamed with visible pus.

Cysts—a severe form of inflammatory acne, cysts are closed hard sacs that can be painful, and are usually treated with prescription drugs.

What Causes Acne?

Acne occurs when androgen hormones cause sebaceous glands to grow and produce excess sebum. The skin cells of the follicle lining shed quickly and in clumps. These cells and increased sebum output are likely to cause clogged pores that become comedones. Finally, acne-causing bacteria which is a normally present on the skin, invades the clogged follicle and begins to multiply rapidly. The result is acne in all of its forms. Retinoids are commonly prescribed for acne prone skin and can make a tremendous difference in the overall appearance of the skin by speeding cell turnover and slowing down oil production. Sometimes two or more acne products are used to treat different acne causes.

What do acne treatments do?

- Reduce sebum production
- Reduce acne causing bacteria
- Normalize the shedding of skin cells

Clearing Up Your Skin

Extraction of comedones should only be performed by a professional under sterile conditions and usually after comedones have not responded to other treatments. While it might be tempting to self-treat blackheads, picking or squeezing blackheads sideways may cause the oil gland to break and aggravate the acne. This can result in inflammation and possible scarring. With appropriate treatment, acne should go away without squeezing.

Regular washing twice a day with a salicylic acid cleanser temporarily helps remove the debris and surface oil that can clog the pores. Toners or astringents containing salicylic acid can also be helpful for oily skin. Other treatments for blackheads include alpha hydroxy acid and salicylic acid peels, which are used as a first defense to prevent cells from building up and clogging pores. Microdermabrasion is also useful to remove surface blackheads.

Over-the-Counter Acne Fighters

A mainstay of over-the-counter acne treatment and a medication commonly prescribed to treat mild forms of acne is benzoyl peroxide. Benzoyl peroxide was the first agent proven to be effective in the treatment of mild acne. It works by killing bacteria on the skin and decreasing sebum. Available over-the-counter in a lotion or a gel, its principal side effect is excessive dryness of the skin.

Salicylic acid helps to correct the abnormal shedding of cells. For milder acne, salicylic acid helps to unclog pores and to prevent new lesions. It must be used continuously, like benzoyl peroxide, since pores will clog up if it is discontinued. Sulfur, in combination with other agents such as alcohol, salicylic acid, and resorcinol, is commonly found in over-the-counter acne preparations. Resorcinol is used with sulfur as well.

Topical Antibiotics

Topical antibiotics are often used in combination with other topical agents. Azelaic acid, a naturally occurring acid, has been adapted for acne treatment in a cream form. Erythromycin is active against a broad spectrum of bacteria. A combination of erythromycin and benzoyl peroxide maximizes the effects of the two and reduces skin oiliness. Clindamycin and tetracycline are also used topically. Sodium sulfonamide lotion is also available for the treatment of acne and for reduction of inflammatory lesions.

Topical Retinoids

Retinoids are very potent anti-acne medications that normalize abnormal growth and reduce dead cell residue in the follicle. Retinoids are available in both topical and systemic forms. The systemic form, isotretinoin or Accutane®, is usually reserved for the most severe acne that is resistant to other treatments. The most common side effects of topical retinoids are redness, dryness, peeling, and itching of skin where the retinoid is applied.

Common topical retinoids:

- **Tretinoin (Retin-A®)** — influences skin cell growth and death cycles. Topical tretinoin is available as a cream, gel or solution

- **Adapalene®** — a synthetic retinoid applied as a gel or cream that has potent anti-inflammatory activity

- **Tazarotene (Tazarac®)** — a synthetic retinoid applied as a gel or cream for acne lesions

Isotretinoin

The gold-standard of acne therapy, particularly for cystic acne, is isotretinoin (Accutane®). It can be extremely effective in treating most forms of acne. Remission for many months to many years is possible. The most common side effect of isotretinoin is dryness of the skin and mucous membranes. Other less common side effects include nausea and vomiting, bone and joint pain, headache, thinning hair, depression, and changes in blood and liver enzyme profiles, which are monitored in regular follow-up examinations. For most men, the possible side effects are worth the benefits of having clear skin.

Oral Medications

A broad-spectrum of antibiotics has been a mainstay in the treatment of moderate to severe, persistent acne for many years. Oral antibiotics treat acne by physiologically affecting the sebaceous follicle and reducing bacterial populations in the follicle. Oral tetracycline has a long history in treating acne and remains one of the most widely used medications. Long-term, low-dose tetracycline therapy may be continued for many months to maintain suppression of acne. Higher doses may be prescribed for very severe acne, with regular monitoring for side effects. Oral erythromycin is an alternative to tetracycline. Minocycline and doxycycline are synthetically derived from tetracycline and both have a long history of use in treating acne.

Light Treatments

The latest treatment for acne is the use of laser and light systems in place of drugs to destroy the bacteria that cause acne. New devices emit a narrow band spectrum of intense light directly onto the skin. Light rays convert a substance produced by acne bacteria into an acne-killing compound. Other forms of non-invasive laser treatments deliver energy down into the oil-producing centers of the sebaceous glands to destroy these oil reservoirs without harming the outer layers of the skin. These lasers work for cystic acne as an alternative to oral and topical medications. Treatments take up to fifteen minutes and may be repeated as needed, once or twice per week for up to eight weeks. In many cases, acne can be controlled for several months at a time. Results may be seen after one treatment. Light therapy can also speed up the healing of active lesions, reduce inflammation, and improve or prevent acne scars.

THE REDNESS OF ROSACEA

"To reduce the severity and occurrences of redness, fragile skin requires vital nutrients to help strengthen cell function, reduce inflammation, and avoid irritation. What is most important is to provide skin with agents that will calm and soothe current symptoms and treat and prevent future eruptions."—Dr. Howard Murad

Rosacea is a chronic disorder that can show up on the cheeks, chin, nose and central forehead. Rosacea is often characterized by remissions and exacerbations. Rosacea appears to be quite common. It has been most frequently observed in men with fair skin, but has also been diagnosed in Asians and African Americans. Rosacea may occur at any age, the onset typically begins after age thirty.

The presence on the face of one or more of the following signs usually indicates rosacea. Rosacea signs come and go, and each may occur independently.

Signs of Rosacea

1. Frequent blushing or flushing

2. Persistent redness of the facial skin

3. Dome-shaped red papules or nodules

4. Broken blood vessels

5. Skin thickening and a bulbous appearance to the tip of the nose (called Rhinophyma), which is more common in men

ITCH FACTOR

Aid for Eczema & Psoriasis

Eczema is a general term that describes various inflamed skin conditions that effect all age groups. It often affects men with a family history of allergies. The severity of the disease can vary. In mild forms the skin is dry, hot, and itchy, while in more severe forms the skin can become broken, raw, and bleed. With treatment, eczema inflammations can be reduced, though the skin will always be sensitive to flare-ups and need extra care. One of the most common forms of eczema is *atopic dermatitis*. In general, *atopic dermatitis* will come and go, often based on external factors. Although its cause is unknown, the condition appears to be an abnormal response of the body's immune system. In men with eczema, the inflammatory response to irritating substances is overactive, causing itching and scratching. Eczema is not contagious and, like many diseases, does not have a definitive cure. However, for most men it can be managed well with treatment and avoidance of triggers.

Although eczema may look different from man to man, it is most often characterized by dry, red, extremely itchy patches on the skin. Eczema is sometimes referred to as "the itch that rashes," since the itch, when scratched, results in the appearance of the rash. Eczema can occur on just about any part of the body. In adults, eczema typically occurs on the face, neck, and the insides of the elbows, knees, and ankles. Chronic scratching causes the skin to take on a leathery texture because the skin has thickened. Many substances have been identified as itch "triggers" and these are not the same for every man. It can be difficult to identify the exact trigger that causes a flare-up. Rough or coarse materials that touch the skin may cause itchiness. Feeling too hot and/or sweating may also cause an outbreak. Other men find that certain soaps, detergents, disinfectants, contact with juices from fresh fruits and meats, dust mites, animal saliva, and hair may trigger itching. Stress can also sometimes aggravate an existing flare-up.

Atopic eczema is thought to be a hereditary condition. Men with atopic eczema are sensitive to allergens in the environment that are harmless to others. Associated conditions include asthma and hayfever. Other types of eczema are caused by contact with irritants such as chemicals and detergents, allergens such as nickel, and yeast growths. As men age, eczema can be caused by circulatory problems in the legs. Adult seborrhoeic eczema is usually seen on the scalp as mild dandruff, but can spread to the face, ears, and chest. The skin becomes red, and inflamed and starts to flake. The condition is believed to be caused by a yeast growth. If the condition becomes infected, treatment with an anti-fungal cream may be necessary.

Eczema is a highly individualized condition, however, the discomfort and distress associated with it can be minimized with an effective skin-care routine, topical creams, and oral steroids, as well as changing the environment. What works for one man will not always work for another. A key to the management of eczema is to prevent scratching. Because eczema is usually dry and itchy, lotions or creams are often prescribed to keep the skin as moist as possible. These are generally most effective when applied within three minutes after bathing to lock in the moisture from the bath. Cold compresses applied directly to itchy skin can also help relieve itching. Skin affected by eczema may frequently become infected because of scratching. Topical or oral antibiotics can kill the bacteria causing the infection.

Anti-Itch Solutions

With flare-ups or when the skin becomes inflamed, steroids are prescribed to reduce inflammation. Topical steroids come in four different strengths: mild, moderately potent, potent, and very potent. The strength of the steroid cream used depends on the severity of the condition, the size of the area, and the part of the body to be treated. Topical steroids are applied thinly to the affected area. Reported side effects such as thinning skin have largely been a result of using very potent steroid preparations over long periods of time. Nonprescription corticosteroid creams and ointments are available for less severe cases. Oral steroids are sometimes prescribed in very severe cases when topical steroids are ineffective.

For severe itching, sedative antihistamines are sometimes used to reduce the itch and are available in both prescription and over-the-counter varieties. Because drowsiness is a common side effect, antihistamines are often used in the evening to help a man restless from eczema get to sleep. Tar treatments and phototherapy are also used and can have positive effects, but tar can be messy. Phototherapy requires special equipment (lights).

Topical immunomodulators (TIMs) are a relatively new class of drugs for the treatment of eczema. TIMs such as Tacrolimus® are topical drugs that modulate the immune response (alter the reactivity of cell-surface immunologic responsiveness). Studies have shown that this class of drugs will improve or completely clear eczema in more than 80 percent of patients.

When eczema is under control, emollients can be used on a daily basis to keep it in check. Emollients are necessary to reduce water loss from the skin, preventing the dryness normally associated with eczema. By providing a seal or barrier, the skin is less dry, and itchy and more comfortable. Emollients are safe to use as often as necessary and are available in various forms: ointments for very dry skin, creams and lotions for mild to moderate or 'wet' eczema. Some are applied directly to the skin, while others are used as soap substitutes.

Eczema can also be controlled by changing behavior. Cotton clothing and sheets keep the skin cool and allow it to breathe, whereas synthetic fabrics and wool can irritate the skin. Using non-biological detergents and avoiding fabric softeners can also help to reduce the itchiness of the skin. Because atopic eczema could be affected by allergens in the droppings of house dust mites, vacuuming and dusting frequently is often recommended.

The following suggestions may help to reduce the severity and frequency of eczema flare-ups:

- Moisturize frequently

- Avoid sudden changes in temperature or humidity

- Avoid sweating or overheating

- Manage stress

- Avoid scratchy materials (e.g., wool or other irritants)

- Avoid harsh soaps, detergents and solvents

- Avoid environmental factors that trigger allergies (e.g., pollens, molds, mites and animal dander)

- Avoid any foods that may cause an outbreak

PSORIASIS

Psoriasis often appears between the ages of fifteen and thirty-five, but it can develop at any age. An inherited disease, it occurs when something triggers the immune system to send a faulty signal to speed up the growth cycle of skin cells. Possible triggers include injury to the skin, stress, infection, and reaction to certain drugs. Once the disease is triggered, the skin cells pile up on the surface of the body faster than normal. In men without psoriasis, skin cells mature and are shed about every twenty-eight days. In psoriatic skin, the skin cells move rapidly up to the surface of the skin over three to six days. The body cannot shed the skin cells fast enough, and this process results in patches forming on the skin's surface.

Psoriasis frequently appears as patches of raised red skin covered by a flaky white buildup found on the knees, elbows, scalp, finger nails, toe nails, and lower back, and less frequently on the palms of the hands, soles of the feet, skin folds of the armpits, groin, buttocks, and on the genitals. It can cause intense itching and burning and painful drying, cracking, or blistering of the skin. Plaque psoriasis can range from mild to severe, and can appear on any skin surface, although the knees, elbows, scalp, trunk, and nails are the most common locations.

Psoriasis is measured in terms of its physical and emotional impact. Physically, if less then 2 percent of the body is involved, the case is considered mild. Between 3 and ten percent is considered moderate, and more than 10 percent is severe. (The palm of one hand equals 1 percent.) Psoriasis is also measured by its impact on quality of life. When psoriasis involves the hands and feet, it may also be considered severe because of how it affects a man's ability to function.

For most men, the symptoms of psoriasis come and go. The time between relapses (episodes of psoriasis) varies greatly. Some men relapse within weeks or months, others go years between episodes.

Treatment for Psoriasis

Psoriasis has no cure, but a wide range of treatments can give men control over this disease. Treatments include the use of skin creams (anthralin, calcipotriene, coal tar, salicyclic acid, steroids, tazarotene); light therapy (lasers: pulse dye and excimer, PUVA, sunlight, ultraviolet light B or UVB); systemic medications in the form of pills or injections (biologics, cyclosporine, methotrexate, oral retinoids); and biologic treatments. The type of psoriasis, its location on the body, its severity, and the patient's age and medical history will determine which treatment is best. The traditional approach is to start with the least potent treatments (topical formulas, phototherapy) and move to stronger ones (such as methotrexate or biologics). The goal is to find a treatment that has the best results and the least amount of side effects.

SKIN TYPES			
SKIN TYPE	**TEXTURE**	**APPEARANCE**	**AGING EFFECTS**
Normal	Equal balance of water and oil, springs back easily	Well-moisturized, medium-sized pores	Age-appropriate lines and wrinkles
Oily	Coarse because oil retains dead skin cells in the hair follicles	Oily areas tend to shine, larger pores	Acne for teenagers and overgrown oil glands in middle and late years
Dry	Rough, flaky texture	Tends to look dull, easily chapped	More likely to become wrinkled as dry skin ages
Combination	Mixture of dry and oily areas	T-zone is most prone to oil while cheeks and neck are dry	Most men have combination skin

DANGERS OF SMOKING

Smoking damages the appearance of the skin. Cigarette smoke and tar deprive the skin of the nutrients and oxygen it needs for good health, ultimately leaving it looking dull and lifeless. Smoking leads to the formation of harmful free radicals and weaken the collagen and elastin fibers, causing the skin to become prematurely wrinkled. The nicotine in smoke narrows the blood vessels, so there is diminished blood supply to the skin.

SKINCARE SOLUTIONS

Men have unique skincare needs and the skincare industry is very well aware of these needs. Products made especially for men are perfume-free, color-free, non-greasy, calming, anti-stress, rinse off easily, and protect the skin. In addition, men also prefer products in packaging that can be quickly sprayed, plastic tubes with flip top lids, or simple containers that travel and pack easily for gym bags and business trips. Men are less inclined to purchase products such as emollient creams, peel-off masks, glass jars with detachable lids, and any kind of product that requires mixing components immediately before application. In short, men want simple, quick, and easy skincare.

SKIN RESURFACING

PEELS

A peel treatment consists of the application of a chemical exfoliating solution to the skin, which peels away the damaged skin and allows new skin to regenerate in its place. Depending on the severity of the skin damage, the solutions are applied in varying concentrations to alter the superficial, medium, or deep layers of the skin. Superficial chemical peels, often referred to as lunchtime peels, remain the cornerstone of any skin rejuvenation program because they require virtually no downtime and produce good results for early signs of aging. The new approaches to chemical peeling using a combination of peeling solutions can maximize results while minimizing side effects. In addition, chemical peeling agents are currently being used to rejuvenate areas other than the face, such as the neck, chest, and hands.

UPDATE ON LASER TECHNOLOGIES

Until recently, there have been two primary categories of laser skin treatment: ablative resurfacing and nonablative laser or light-based therapy, each with their advantages and disadvantages. Ablative techniques can effectively rejuvenate aging and sun-damaged skin but have significant side effects, risks, and prolonged healing and recovery times. Nonablative techniques generally carry fewer risks but require numerous treatments over several months, producing variable improvement.

FRACTIONAL RESURFACING TECHNOLOGY

Unlike ablative lasers that remove the top layer of skin, the Fraxel® laser treatment produces tiny, microscopic sites of thermal impact separated by areas of healthy tissue. At the same time, the energy penetrates the dermis to remodel collagen. The Fraxel® laser is specially designed to alter only fractional volumes of the target tissue. After cleansing with a mild cleanser, a blue tint (OptiGuide Blue) is applied to the skin. Then, a topical anesthetic ointment is applied to the treatment area. The blue tint darkens the tiny folds of the skin surface to increase contrast and allows a robotic hand piece to precisely read the contours of the treatment area as it glides across the skin. The blue tint and anesthetic are washed off immediately after treatment. A treatment typically takes approximately 30 -45 minutes for the full face and neck. Side effects typically involve some swelling and redness, peeling and flaking for several days. Four treatments are recommended to produce a gradual tissue remodeling that improves over time.

LED Technology

Photomodulation refers to using low-energy light to accelerate or inhibit cell activity. Unlike laser technology that relies on high-powered light to create heat energy, LED photomodulation triggers the body and the chemical to convert light energy into cell energy without using heat. The treatment is both painless and quick, (lasting only thirty-six seconds) with no downtime. When this light shines on the skin in a specific pulsing repetition, the enzyme that is responsible for collagen breakdown will decrease, therefore increasing the total amount of collagen in the skin. One treatment per week for eight weeks, followed by maintenance treatments, result in a clearer skin texture with a reduction of fine lines and a more even complexion. It may also be used in conjunction with other procedures such as microdermabrasion to enhance the results. LED devices are also being used after deeper treatments to speed up the healing process and reduce downtime.

RADIO FREQUENCY SKIN TIGHTENING

There are several radio frequency systems currently on the market, and more under development. The most well known is Thermage®. The treatment uses a handheld instrument to transmit an electric radio frequency through the skin to heat the collagen fibers in the dermis causing them to contract and tighten. It stimulates the growth of new collagen over several months, which further firms the skin. While the pulses of energy are being delivered, a cryogen cooling spray keeps the surface of the skin from burning. The Thermage® procedure is also being used to treat areas of the body including droopy buttocks and slackened elbows and knees. For early signs of aging, a radiofrequency procedure may be used to subtly tighten the lower face and neck. The treatment can be as short as twenty-five minutes for the brow area, and forty-five minutes for the full face in one session. One may feel an intense prickling sensation, and for most men, a topical numbing cream is needed. Results are not immediate, but may improve over the course of two to five months as the skin becomes firmer. One or more treatments may be needed. This technology is also good for acne scars.

PIGMENT PROBLEM SOLVERS

In the young, they are called freckles. As one gets older, they are called age spots. Hyperpigmentation simply means an excess of pigment in the skin. If a patient feels like his complexion is being punished by unsightly brown patches that never seem to go away, he is not alone. Hyperpigmentation is the result of overly abundant production of melanin in the epidermis, associated with sun exposure, injury, and infection.

Pigmented skin can be difficult to treat, but new options continue to be introduced. Advances in treatment include a combination therapy of topical formulas alongside more aggressive medical treatments and maintenance for best results. As with any other skin condition, the key to managing hyperpigmentation is long-term total sun avoidance.

The first step in the treatment of hyperpigmentation is to determine the cause. A complete medical history and a proper physical examination including an evaluation of the skin will be performed. Diagnostic tests, including thyroid function tests and skin biopsies, may be appropriate. The next step is to eliminate the cause, if possible. For example, if the cause is medication, discontinuing it may result in an improvement.

Dark patches tend to darken in summer after sun exposure, and fade in winter when the sun is less strong. This happens because the skin's pigment, or melanin, absorbs the energy of the sun's UV rays in order to protect the skin from overexposure. Tanning occurs as a result, causing dark areas to get even darker. Skin inflammations from allergic reactions or acne can also be a trigger.

1. Genetic factors
2. Thyroid dysfunction
3. Certain medications
4. Nutritional deficiencies

Melanocytes are the cells in the epidermis that produce melanin. They respond to sunlight by producing more melanin to protect the keratinocytes (one of the main reasons for melanin production). UV light also causes an inflammation of the skin. The long-term effects of solar radiation will cause pigment to pool from leaking melanocytes. This phenomenon produces age spots. In this case, the melanocyte has been damaged by UV exposure and needs to be repaired.

With injury or infection, a red papule is formed that eventually turns into a hyperpigmented spot. This is due to increased melanocyte activity, which produces more melanin in response to inflammation. In a normal situation, when the inflammation subsides, the resulting hyperpigmentation sloughs off as the cell moves to the top of the epidermis.

Tyrosinase is an enzyme that determines just how much melanin is produced. The majority of products available to treat hyperpigmentation inhibit tyrosinase in one way or another. Hydroquinone is still widely considered the most effective skin-lightening agent. Hydroquinone has been considered the gold standard for effective reduction of hyperpigmentation. It can slow down or stop production of melanin in many conditions, such as post-inflammatory hyperpigmentation. Hydroquinone should be discontinued if no improvements occur within four to six months due to the potential risks of long-term use.

DARKER SKIN TYPES

Men with darker skin have different complexion issues. These skin types are pigment protected so they do not burn as easily as fair complexions, but they are at greater risk for discoloration and melasma. On the Fitzpatrick skin scale of I to VI, skin types III and higher have special needs that are not always adequately addressed by the cosmetics and skincare treatments commercially available.

An African American or Asian man at age fifty, compared to a blonde, blue-eyed European of the same age who has been exposed to the sun, will typically have better facial elasticity and look younger. Delayed wrinkling is related to higher melanin production which provides natural sun protection. The downside is that bronze skin tends to darken before it burns, and can develop chronic hyperpigmentation earlier. In my practice, the major skin concern for dark brown to black complexions is discoloration.

Post-inflammatory hyperpigmentation is a widespread problem. Men with darker skin tones often experience discoloration from a variety of causes such as acne, insect bites, scratches, eczema, chicken pox scars, abrasions, or overexposure to the sun. Picking the skin has a tendency to leave deep scars and discoloration that usually appears darker than the rest of the skin. Areas that are more prone to discoloration include the joints (knees, elbows, and ankles) and eyelid area. The problem of pigmentation in patients with darker skin is further complicated by the fact that darker skin types do not always respond well to resurfacing treatments or procedures that can be used to lighten pigmented areas.

Other special concerns for men with darker skin include ingrown hairs or razor bumps that are caused by excessively close shaving of curly hair (pseudo folliculitis barbae or PFB). Keloids and hypertrophic scars are also more of a risk in darker skin types. Fortunately, hypertrophic scars that are raised and pink are far more common than true keloids. Perhaps the good news is that compared with fair skin types, men with darker and thicker skin are less inclined to need anti-aging treatments such as wrinkle fillers, Botox® injections, and laser resurfacing.

Black Skin—Black skin can be quite sensitive, discolors quickly, and scars easily because of the more active melanocytes. It is much more sensitive to the sun's harmful rays than most people assume, which is a primary cause of the discoloration. Ashy complexions frequently make black skin look blotchy. Shine from excess oil is also a common problem.

Asian Skin—Asian skin can range in complexion from very fair, to more dark olive shades with yellow undertones, and from dry to very oily. The higher concentration of pigmentation a man has, the easier he can scar and discolor. Yellow tinted skin has active pigmentation, which makes it very susceptible to sun damage, scarring, and discoloration. Asian skin tends to be the most transparent and soft, which leads to magnification of every spot and scar.

Latino Skin—Olive and Mediterranean skin types have the firmest skin of the bronze spectrum. The skin is often oily. Firm skin can protect from deep scarring but may also cause many problems for the complexion. Much of the skin turmoil comes from overactive sebaceous glands that bring excess oil to the skin's surface, causing enlarged pores and blackheads. Firm skin is frequently the cause of ingrown hairs and dark spots from breakouts.

CHAPTER 9

Reversing Sun Damage

Pre-cancerous lesions called Actinic Keratoses affect approximately one in six men.

Because exposure to the sun influences how well the skin ages, protecting the skin from the sun is the single most important practice in skincare. Continuous exposure to the sun will wrinkle and dry out the skin, leaving it coarse and thick. Uneven pigmentation, from freckles to brown spots, is another undesirable side effect. The earliest warning sign of severe skin damage is the development of "actinic keratoses." These precancerous lesions are most common in men with fair skin and light hair, but can occur in any skin type with chronic sun exposure. As a man ages, cumulative sun damage will start to crop up, no matter what. The sun's rays are very unforgiving, and the damage they do to the skin is inescapable.

Sunscreen does not necessarily reduce wrinkles, but consistent use will stop them from forming as quickly and as deeply. It is never too late to begin protecting the skin from the sun.

Preventing Sun Damage

- Avoid unnecessary sun exposure, especially during the sun's peak hours (10 AM to 4 PM) for harmful ultraviolet (UV) radiation
- Cover up with clothing, including a broad-brimmed hat, long pants, a long-sleeved shirt, and UV-blocking sunglasses
- Wear a broad-spectrum sunscreen with a sun protection factor (SPF) 15 or higher. Apply liberally, uniformly and frequently
- Avoid tanning parlors and artificial tanning devices
- Examine skin from head to toe once every month
- Have a skin examination with a dermatologist annually
- Year-round sun protection is critical
- The sun's harmful ultraviolet radiation can penetrate many types of clothes.
- It can also go through automobile and residential windows
- It can damage the eyes, contributing to cataracts, macular degeneration, and eyelid cancers
- When on snow or ice, the face and eyes are at almost twice the risk of UV damage because of reflected glare

Sun Protection Decoded

There is tremendous confusion concerning the differences between various formulations of sunscreen and sun blocks because the terminology of sun protection is often confusing. Sun protection factor is the measure of UVB (not UVA) protection provided from a sunscreen product. For example, SPF 30 provides thirty times more sun protection than skin's natural sunburn protection. SPF 15 blocks out 93 percent of burning UVB rays. SPF 30 blocks out 97 percent of burning UVB rays. There is a difference between sunscreens and sun blocks. The ideal sunscreen will provide you with the necessary level of protection for skin type, degree of sun exposure, and sun sensitivity. SPF ratings are based on how much longer someone may be protected from sunburn than he would be if no sunscreen were applied. For instance, if a man normally burns in twenty minutes, a product with SPF 15 will allow him to stay out in the sun fifteen times longer. One will be able to stay out in the sun without burning for five hours, assuming the sunscreen is applied properly. The SPF number doesn't refer to a sunscreen's strength. For example, an SPF 30 is no stronger than an SPF 8—it does not filter out more harmful rays than an SPF 8 does—but it does protect for longer.

A "sunscreen" shields skin to prevent harmful UVA/UVB rays from penetrating skin. SPF 15 and 30 work this way by absorbing, blocking, deflecting, and scattering UV light. Both contain new transparent zinc oxide. SPF 20 shields skin by absorbing UV light. Products containing Parsol 1789, zinc oxide, or titanium dioxide are the key UVA blockers.

A "very water resistant" sunscreen should be reapplied sixty minutes after swimming or excessive perspiration to maintain its SPF protection. SPF 20 is considered "very water resistant." The term "waterproof" is no longer used since no sunscreen is completely waterproof. Ultraviolet rays are always present—winter, summer, even on cloudy days— so it is vital to be properly protected at all times.

"The ideal sunscreen for you is one that will provide you with the necessary level of protection for your skin type, degree of sun exposure, and risk for sun sensitivity."—Dr. Howard Murad

Whatever the sunscreen of choice, the key is to use enough of it on a regular basis; apply an SPF 15 broad spectrum sunscreen generously every two hours. Most men do not use nearly enough sunscreen to provide adequate coverage. Use a liberal application of one ounce—the equivalent of shot glass—to cover all exposed parts of the body. The higher a product's sun protection factor rating, the stronger and longer its effects will be.

Timing is important, too. Sunscreens need to be applied 30 minutes before getting to the pool or beach, not after arriving. Men who get intense sun exposure during outdoor sports or boating should use more complete coverage in the form of a sun block of SPF 30 or higher. Water resistant lotions have an oil base, which is thicker and heavier, and may clog pores. For oily skin, stick with oil-free formulas that will not make one look and feel shiny or break out. Most men prefer a sunscreen that is water resistant and does not run into the eyes. Even water resistant sunscreens need to be reapplied every 90 minutes.

Medications and Sun Exposure

Many drugs increase sensitivity to sunlight and the risk of getting a sunburn. Some common ones include thiazides, some diuretics, tetracycline and sulfa antibiotics, and nonsteroidal anti-inflammatory drugs such as ibuprofen, in dosages used to treat arthritis.

If a sunburn develops, take aspirin or ibuprofen (Advil, Motrin, others) for pain, apply cold compresses, and avoid further exposure until the burn goes away. A sunburn spray may help relieve pain. A severe sunburn may require medical attention.

Tanning Beds

Avoid tanning beds entirely, as they can cause skin cancer, infections, and warts. We know that UVB and sunburns are associated with increased skin cancer and melanoma risk. UVA radiation may also increase the risk of skin cancer or melanoma.

PRECANCEROUS CONDITIONS

Any man who spends time in the sun runs a high risk of developing one or more actinic keratosis. Also known as a solar keratosis, it is a scaly or crusty bump that arises on the skin's surface. The base may be light or dark, tan, pink, red, a combination of these or the same color as the skin. The scale or crust is horny, dry and rough, and is often recognized by touch rather than sight. Occasionally it itches or produces a pricking or tender sensation. It can also become inflamed and surrounded by redness, and in rare instances, bleed. Early on, it may disappear only to reappear later. Several actinic keratoses are often at a time.

An actinic keratosis is most likely to appear on the face, ears, scalp, neck, backs of the hands and forearms, shoulders and lips—the parts of the body most often exposed to the sun. The growths may be flat and pink or raised and rough. Actinic cheilitis is a type of actinic keratosis occurring on the lips, which causes them to become dry, cracked, scaly, pale, or white. It mainly affects the lower lip, which typically receives more sun exposure than the upper lip.

Actinic keratoses are considered a precursor of cancer, or a pre-cancer. If treated early, almost all actinic keratoses can be eliminated without becoming skin cancers. If left untreated, about 2 to 5 percent of these lesions may progress to squamous cell carcinomas. They can grow large and invade the surrounding tissues. The more keratoses present, the greater the chance that one or more may turn into skin cancer. Any change in a pre-existing skin growth, or the development of a new growth or open sore that fails to heal, should prompt an immediate visit to a physician. In many cases, a simple surgical procedure or application of a topical chemotherapeutic agent may be the only treatment required.

Older men are more likely than younger men to develop these lesions, because cumulative sun exposure increases with the years. Actinic keratoses also appear in men in their early twenties who have spent too much time in the sun with little or no protection. Men may also have up to ten times as many subclinical (invisible) lesions as visible lesions on the surface of the skin. The lighter the skin, the greater risk there is of developing actinic keratoses. However, even darker-skinned men are at risk if they are exposed to the sun without protection.

SKIN CANCER WARNING SIGNS

According to the Skin Cancer Foundation (www.skincancer.org), knowing the warning signs—the ABCDs—of a malignant melanoma can help possible problem areas on the skin.

MALE TALE: Barry, age 46, is a Director of Marketing for a financial services firm. His company orders all their executives to have an annual physical. Two years ago, during a routine check up, he was diagnosed with a melanoma. "My doctor saw something on my shoulder that he didn't like the look of. When he suggested that I see the dermatologist across the hall for a biopsy, I just thought he was being extra cautious," says Barry. One week later, he got the bad news. "I was blown away," he says now, "it was the last thing I expected." Barry was one of the lucky ones. His melanoma was small, in its early stages, and very treatable. A lifetime of summers at Cape Cod without sunscreen had finally caught up with him.

MELANOMA

Melanoma is the most serious form of skin cancer. If it is diagnosed and removed while it is thin and limited to the outermost skin layer, it is almost 100 percent curable. Once the cancer advances and spreads to other parts of the body, it is hard to treat and can be deadly. Melanoma is a malignant tumor that originates in melanocytes, the cells that produce the pigment melanin that colors our skin, hair, and eyes, and is heavily concentrated in most moles. The majority of melanomas, therefore, are black or brown. However, melanomas occasionally stop producing pigment. When that happens, the melanomas may no longer be dark, but are skin-colored, pink, red or purple.

The melanoma may be in early or advanced stages, localized, or invasive. Localized melanomas occupy only the uppermost part of the epidermis, the top layers of the skin. Invasive melanomas are more serious, as they have penetrated more deeply into the skin and may have traveled from the original tumor through the body.

Four Basic Types

Malignant melanomas are usually small brown-black or larger multicolored patches, plaques, or nodules with irregular outline. They may crust on the surface or bleed. Many of them may arise in pre-existing moles.

Superficial spreading melanoma is the most common type, accounting for about 70 percent of all cases. This melanoma travels along the top layer of the skin for a long time before penetrating more deeply. The first sign is the appearance of a flat or slightly raised discolored patch that has irregular borders and is somewhat geometrical in form. The color varies, and areas of tan, brown, black, red, blue, or white may be visible. Sometimes an older mole will change in these ways, or a new one will arise. The melanoma can be seen almost anywhere on the body but is most likely to occur on the trunk and the upper back in men. Most melanomas found in the young are of the superficial spreading type.

Lentigo maligna is similar to the superficial spreading type, as it also remains close to the skin's surface for quite a while, and usually appears as a flat or mildly elevated mottled tan, brown, or dark brown discoloration. This type of localized melanoma is found most often in the elderly on chronically sun-exposed, damaged skin on the face, ears, arms, and upper trunk.

Acral lentiginous melanoma also spreads superficially before penetrating more deeply. It is quite different from the others, though, because it usually appears as a black or brown discoloration under the nails or on

RHINOPLASTY

This thirty-four-year-old musician was teased all his life about his large nose, so he sought to refine his nose without an "overdone" look. The patient underwent cosmetic rhinoplasty and also treatment of internal nasal airway obstruction.

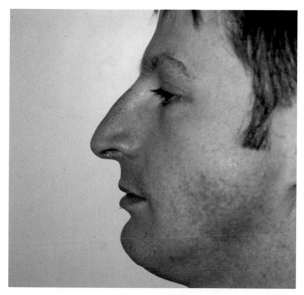

Before

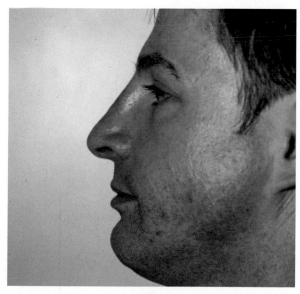

After

LIPOSUCTION OF ABDOMEN AND "LOVE HANDLES"

This thirty-six-year-old physician, despite diet and exercise, could not obtain a desired "chiseled" abdomen. The patient underwent extended liposuction of the entire abdomen and hip rolls.

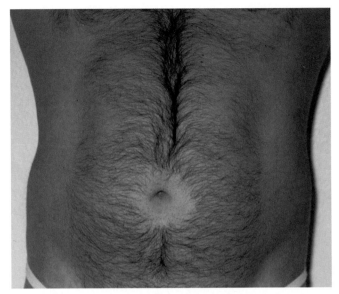

Before (frontal view)

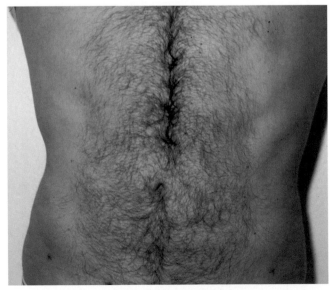

After (frontal view)

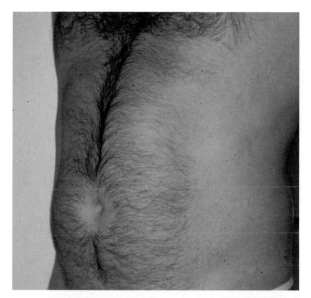

Before (three-quarter view)

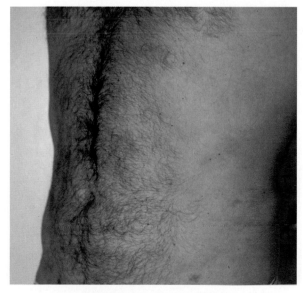

After (three-quarter view)

GYNECOMASTIA

A forty-two-year-old accountant, with gynecomastia since puberty, this man had dieted and exercised to no avail. He desired a flatter, more sculpted chest, which would reveal his well developed underlying musculature. Patient underwent liposuction and open excision of gynecomastia.

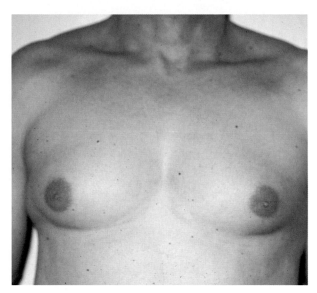

Before (frontal view)

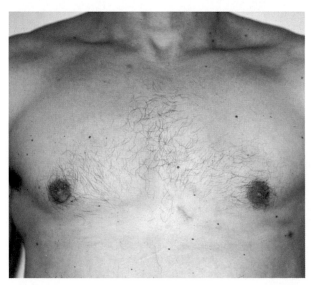

After (frontal view)

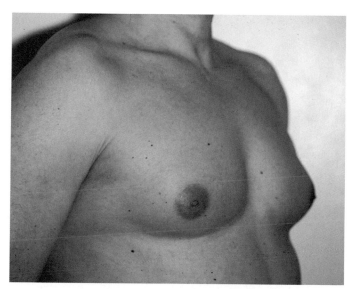

Before (three-quarter view)

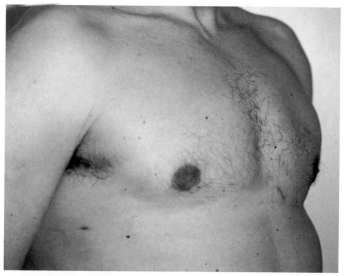

After (three-quarter view)

SKIN FILLER

This fifty-two-year-old teacher complained of hollow cheeks (fat atrophy), which resulted in a "sick look" despite excellent health. His treatment consisted of injections of Sculptra to both cheeks over several months in order to fill in the hollows.

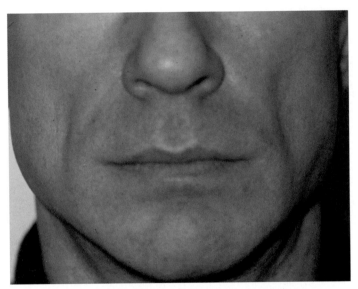

Before (frontal view)

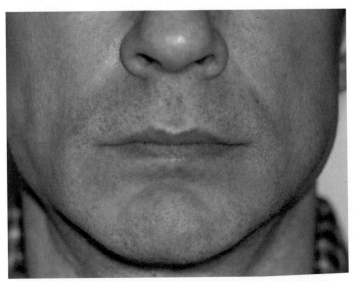

After (frontal view)

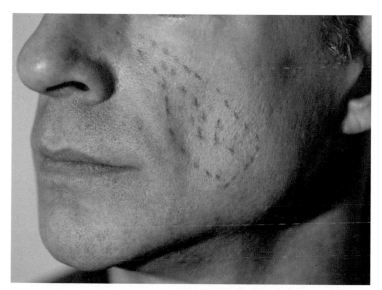

Before (three-quarter view)

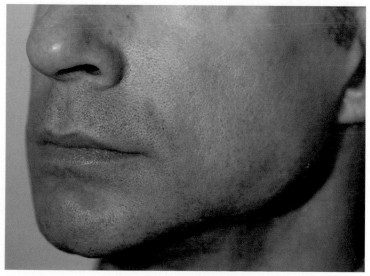

After (three-quarter view)

UPPER AND LOWER EYELIDS AND MIDFACE LIFT

A fifty-seven-year-old actor, this complained of looking tired and haggard in front of the camera. He sought surgery to look more alert but not appear overdone. He underwent conservative upper eyelid tuck and lower eyelid tuck combined with mid-facelift.

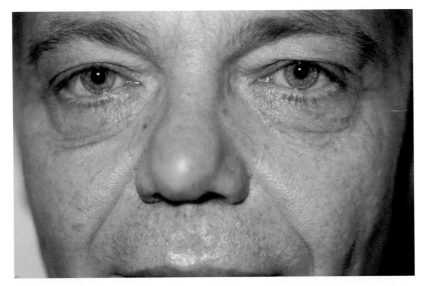

Before

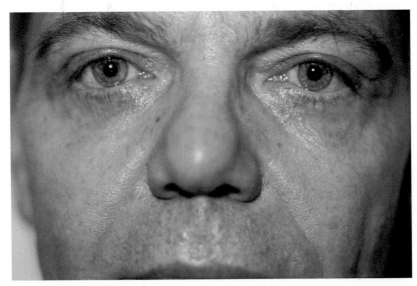

After

the soles of the feet or palms of the hands. This type of melanoma is most often found in dark-skinned men. It is the most common melanoma in African-Americans and Asians and the least common among Caucasians.

Nodular melanoma, unlike the other three types, is usually invasive when it is first diagnosed. The malignancy is recognized when it becomes a bump. The color is most often black but is occasionally blue, gray, white, brown, tan, red, or skin tone. The most frequent locations are the trunk, legs and arms (mainly of elderly men), as well as the scalp in men.

BASAL CELL CARCINOMA

Basal cell carcinoma is the most common form of skin cancer, affecting 800,000 Americans each year. In fact, it is the most common of all cancers. These cancers arise in the basal cells, which are at the bottom of the epidermis (outer skin layer). Until recently, those most often affected were older people, particularly men who had worked outdoors. The number of men with BCC greatly outnumbers women.

Chronic exposure to sunlight is the cause of almost all basal cell carcinomas, which occur most frequently on exposed parts of the body—the face, ears, neck, scalp, shoulders, and back. Tumors may also develop on non-exposed areas. In rare cases, contact with arsenic, exposure to radiation, and complications of burns, scars, vaccinations, or even tattoos are contributing factors.

Anyone with a history of frequent sun exposure can develop basal cell carcinoma. Men who have fair skin, light hair, and blue, green, or gray eyes are at the highest risk. Those whose occupations require long hours outside or who spend extensive leisure time in the sun are in particular jeopardy. Dark-skinned individuals are far less likely than those who are fair-skinned to develop skin cancer.

Learn the signs of basal cell carcinoma, and examine the skin regularly—as often as once a month if at high risk. Be sure to include the scalp, backs of ears, neck, and other hard-to-see areas. (A full-length mirror and a hand-held mirror can be very useful). If any of the warning signs or some other change in the skin are visible, consult a dermatologist immediately.

SQUAMOUS CELL

Squamous cell carcinoma, the second most common skin cancer after basal cell carcinoma, arises from the epidermis. Squamous cell cancers may occur on all areas of the body including the mucous membranes (i.e. lips), but are most common in areas exposed to the sun.

Although squamous cell carcinomas usually remain confined to the epidermis for some time, they eventually penetrate the underlying tissues if they are not treated. In a small percentage of cases, they spread (metastasize) to distant tissues and organs. When this happens, they can be fatal.

Squamous cell carcinomas occur most frequently on areas of the body that have been exposed to the sun for prolonged periods. That is why tumors appear most frequently on sun-exposed parts of the body: the face, neck, bald scalp, hands, shoulders, arms, and back. The rim of the ear and the lower lip are especially vulnerable to the development of these cancers. Squamous cell carcinomas may also occur where skin has suffered certain kinds of injury: burns, scars, long-standing sores, and sites previously exposed to X-rays.

Men with light hair and coloring are also most at risk for this type of cancer, as are those who spend a great deal of time outside in direct sunlight.

Warning Signs of Squamous Cell Carcinoma

- A wart-like growth that crusts and occasionally bleeds

- A persistent, scaly red patch with irregular borders that sometimes crusts or bleeds. An open sore that bleeds, crusts and persists for weeks

- An elevated growth with a central depression that occasionally bleeds. A growth of this type may rapidly increase in size

A Word to the Wise

Sun damage to the skin accumulates over time, so even a brief exposure adds to the lifetime total. The likelihood of developing actinic keratosis is highest in regions near the equator. However, regardless of climate, every man is exposed to the sun. About 80 percent of solar UV rays can pass through clouds. These rays can also bounce off sand, snow, sidewalks, and other reflective surfaces, giving extra exposure.

Topical Medications

Medicated creams and solutions are especially useful in removing both visible and invisible actinic keratoses when the lesions are numerous. Medication is applied according to a schedule worked out by a doctor. After treatment, some discomfort may result from skin breakdown. 5-fluorouracil (5-FU) cream or solution, in concentrations from 0.5 to 5 percent, is the most widely used topical treatment for actinic keratoses. It works especially well on the face, ears, and neck. Some swelling and crusting may occur. Imiquod cream is also being used for multiple keratoses. It causes cells to produce interferon, a chemical that destroys cancerous and precancerous cells.

New and improved treatments are constantly under development, and it is wise to have a full body check with a dermatologist at least annually, and every six months if a history of skin cancer is present.

CHAPTER 10

Hair, Hands & Feet

"A style should reflect one's personality, lifestyle, and individual taste, not necessarily the latest trends. I always advise my clients to choose a style they can maintain and one they are comfortable and confident wearing." —Frédéric Fekkai

Exposure to UV rays has the same effect on hair as it does on the skin. The physical changes include the destruction of cuticle cells, roughening of the hair surface, loss of elastic strength, and increased absorption of moisture. Those with a darker hair color have more melanin, and will show more damage. Lifeguards typically have light streaks running through their hair that give it a dry, straw-like appearance. Any harsh, natural condition can have a negative effect on the quality and strength of hair. When the hair is damaged, dirt and other particles can become lodged between the scales, which make hair look dull. Gray hair is particularly susceptible to damage from the sun, which can give it a yellowish tint.

THE ENEMY	HAIR PROTECTION
Salt water	Rinse or wash hair after swimming in an ocean
Sun exposure	Wear hat; spray hair with styling product with SPF
Steam heat	Use humidifier at night; conditioning hair weekly
Chlorinated pools	Wash hair immediately after swimming
Extreme temperatures	Wear hats to keep hair covered
Wind	Wear cap
Pollution	Use spray with SPF, use clarifying products

CLEAN REGIME

Just like the face, the hair needs a ritual for morning, night, and emergencies that can change with the seasons. Healthy-looking hair starts in the shower. Go gentle on the follicles to maintain as many hairs as possible for as long as possible. Too much cleansing, pulling, tugging, and styling makes hair more brittle and keeps it weak. Every shampoo bottle has directions to shampoo twice before rinsing. In theory, the first rinse removes dirt, oil, and product buildup, and the second lather helps add volume. It also serves as a backup in case the first shampoo does not clean the hair thoroughly enough. For dry or brittle hair, one shampoo may be enough. With airborne pollutants, holes in the ozone layer, and steam heat, the hair tends to attract dust and dirt.

For some men, daily washing with a shampoo formulated to restore balance to both the hair and scalp is a necessity. Some guys are happy to skip a day or two. For short hair, daily washing is usually needed. Washing hair more than once a day is not necessary or recommended. The hair produces natural oils each day, which provide thickness and shine. Over-washing will strip these oils away.

Between work, play, and social obligations most men do not have the time or patience to primp. For men on the go, celebrity stylist Frédéric Fekkai offers the three golden rules to get the most mileage from the hair:

• Go for a haircut every 4–6 weeks to keep hair looking shiny and healthy

• Be sure to use the appropriate shampoo for hair type. If the scalp is dry and irritated, use shampoo created to treat that (i.e. Fekkai Sensitive Scalp Shampoo)

• Limit the amount of styling product used each application. A little goes a long way, to avoid hair that looks greasy and overdone

5-STEP CLEANSING

1. Get the full head of hair wet before shampooing. Thoroughly saturated hair builds a better lather, so use less shampoo for cleaner hair

2. Use a minimal amount of mild shampoo, only as often as necessary to keep hair clean

3. Rinse thoroughly twice to make sure to remove all shampoo residue. Squeeze excess water out hair before using conditioner

4. Apply only a small dollop of conditioner, starting at the ends first and working up. Conditioner is rarely needed on the scalp and tends to weigh hair down

5. Immediately after applying conditioner, use a wide tooth comb to spread it evenly throughout your hair. Hair is three times weaker when it is wet.

Oil Control

Oily hair may be greasy at the scalp, but dull at the ends. Fine, thin hair is the most prone to looking oily and limp. To prevent oil buildup, wash hair daily using a mild shampoo without conditioner to minimize the amount of residue. Formulas specifically designed for oily hair, or clarifying shampoos work well. Use a very light cream rinse or conditioner or a diluted formula only on the ends and rinse out thoroughly. Avoid products that contain silicone, oils, or lanolin. If the hair becomes stringy by the middle of the day, spray some water on your hair and comb through to remove and redistribute oils. In humid weather, take showers daily and wash hair more often, especially if it is oily. Switch to a gentle shampoo specifically designed for frequent use. For those who exercise often and sweat a lot, shampoo after working out too.

The Shampoo Jungle

Selecting the right products will help make the most of the hair. It is important to use the right gel or spray specifically formulated for hair type. As the hair's texture or thickness changes, update the products used to achieve the desired look you want.

An effective shampoo removes all traces of dirt and excess oil from the hair and cleans the scalp by removing the top layer of dead skin cells. Most shampoos contain either soap-based or synthetic detergents. Soap-based shampoos work as an active cleanser, but they can leave residue. On the other hand, synthetic detergents do not leave a residue; the strength of the detergent determines if the shampoo is suitable for dry, normal, or oily hair. Acid is often added to shampoo to balance the alkalinity that leaves hair looking dull. Conditioners that are added to shampoos often counteract the detergent and make two-in-one shampoos less effective. Medicated shampoos address skin-related scalp problems, such as dandruff or psorasis by slowing the growth of skin cells and controlling oil glands on the scalp.

The best shampoos for hair should be at a pH of 4.5 to 6, which is closest to the natural pH of the scalp and hair.

All-in-one shampoo and conditioners—They may seem practical and economical, but shampoo-conditioner combos tend to build up quickly, and they weigh down hair. They should never be used on oily hair. They are best reserved for travel.

Volumizing shampoos—These contain proteins that bond to the hair to add volume, strand by strand. Use them sparingly. If they are overused, they can build up a residue. For fine hair, alternate with a regular shampoo. Look for ingredients like 'dimethicone copolyol,' a silicon derivative that helps build volume in hair. Wash hair regularly, as the static electricity from clean hair naturally boosts volume.

Time to switch shampoos?

- The hair looks better the morning after washing
- The hair feels weighed down, needs to be rinsed more
- The hair is difficult to style
- The hair does not look shiny
- Sudsing does not give a rich lather anymore

Hair Conditioning

Conditioners make the hair smoother and add body and shine, but there is a delicate balance between the right amount and over conditioning. Conditioners are usually made of large molecules that literally stick to the outside of the hair and make combing easier, which prevents the hair from twisting and breaking. Hair tangles when the cuticle does not lie flat and the hairs cannot slide by one another with ease. Because they coat the hair, conditioners make it look shiny and protect it from damage from the environment and styling tools. They contain silicone and humectants such as ceramides and complex lipids that smooth over hair and can reduce frizz and static electricity. Although conditioners can add thickness and volume to thinning hair, over-conditioning may cause hair to look greasy. It can cause the cuticle layer of the hair to lift, making hair brittle and easily broken. For thinning hair, use only lightweight, rinse-out conditioners or cream rinses. Volumizers with ingredients such as keratin, collagen, and hydrolyzed proteins are helpful to plump up strands to make hair look fuller. Conditioners should be at a low pH of 4.0 to 4.5 to maintain the protein in the hair.

Rinse-out conditioners—Increase shine, smooth the hair cuticle, soften the hair, reduce static. Used after shampooing, and rinsed out thoroughly. Good for most hair types.

Leave-in conditioners—Usually applied to towel-dried hair that gets blown dry often. These formulas coat the hair, so they can make hair heavier and weigh it down. Some formulas have UV protection built in to protect hair from sun, wind, and heat.

Thickening Serums—Make hair appear fuller, bind proteins and polymers to the hair shaft. Applied before styling on wet or dry hair.

Holding Patterns

Styling products add shine and texture and to control flyaway hairs.

Gels or fixatives—Look for gels that offer thickening, light, or medium hold, designed for fine or thinning hair. A light gel can help add body and volume to the hair, but stay away from thick, goopy gels that weigh hair down.

Sprays—If the hair is extremely thin or limp, try a fine misting spray instead of gel. Stiff hairsprays will make hair sticky.

Mousse—Good as a styling aid because they are light and foamy, but as with all hair products for thin hair, less is more.

A good rule of thumb when purchasing a hair product is to avoid formulas that contain alcohol. It can be drying on the scalp and skin, says Frédéric Fekkai.

Tool Time

What is used in the hair is as critical as what is put on it. Styling tools can break, split, and damage the cuticle, which can accentuate hair loss. Use only wide-tooth combs; polished wood or tortoise shell is preferred. The next best thing would be hard rubber. Avoid using metal or cheap, flimsy combs made of plastic or rubber, or any combs that have jagged teeth.

Frédéric Fekkai encourages his male clients to buy a treatment comb and to have grooming clay or gel on hand—like Fekkai Men's Grooming Clay or Fekkai For Men Hair. They keep hair styled and in place throughout the day.

Caring for Your Combs

Like the scalp, the comb suffers from oily build up and product overload.

* Remove hairs from in between teeth after use
* Wash combs weekly in warm soapy water
* Carefully dry teeth thoroughly

BARBER VS STYLIST

Finding the right stylist is like dating: it is a long-term relationship and chemistry counts. Just find the person that does the best scissor work for you. Barbershops are assembly lines for haircuts. The less hair, the more logical this choice, especially to keep simple and short. If unsure about the look—or if you want something specific—a barber is more likely to disappoint. Stylists will take more time to create a cut that will work. They usually charge a lot more than a barber too. Communication is important, and it may take time to get to know each other and get it right. A good stylist will keep hair looking good as he grows accustomed to your hair's particular habits. Hair should be trimmed on a regular basis, approximately every six weeks.

Hair comes in three basic textures determined by the diameter or thickness of the strands:

- **Fine**—50 microns—only about 15 percent have it
- **Medium**—60-90 microns—most common
- **Coarse**—100 microns +

Fine hair

- It is often wavy, but rarely curly
- It can look stringy and limp when it gets longer
- It often hangs flat and lies close to the head
- It looks thin even if there is a lot of it
- It has a silkier feel

Coarse hair

- It is stronger and sturdier
- Often appears bushy or wiry in humidity
- Tends to look dull even after it is just washed
- Needs constant conditioning
- When it is curly, it tends to be dry on the top layers
- When it is straight, it retains water easily

The number of hairs on the head determines whether the hair is thick or thin. Hair strands can be as thin as 1/1,000 of an inch, and as thick as 1/140 of an inch.

Volumizers

- Wash hair regularly so that the static electricity from clean hair naturally boosts the volume
- For straight hair, blow dry with a boar-bristle brush
- For curly hair, blow dry with a diffuser attachment

Dry hair is relative. Insufficient moisture and oil will make hair look dry. Dry, brittle hair may also be the result of excessive washing, harsh detergents, heat processing, and a dry or hostile environment. One way to combat the coarse, brittle look and texture of dry hair is with conditioner. If the hair is on the dry side, use a conditioner after every shampoo for softer, shinier hair. However, even conditioners cannot really revitalize or fix severely damaged hair. If it is constantly dry and intensive conditioning does not seem to help, see a doctor. Fragile hair that breaks easily may be a signal of more than just a problem of vanity. It may be caused by underlying medical conditions, such as metabolic diseases, hypothyroidism, and poor nutrition. Abnormally dry, lifeless hair can also result from the natural oil being stripped from the cuticle, or from dandruff, which can clog the oil glands.

Any tool that adds heat can cause more damage to hair. Use these only on a cool setting. Hair also tends to dry out during winter, if one lives in a cold climate, uses steam heat, or has had a lot of sun exposure.

Damage Control

- Apply a drop of shine-enhancing serum or cream to damp hair

- Air-dry hair whenever possible

- Twice a week, use a cream conditioner applied to the ends and leave on for 20 minutes

- Using a humidifier can replace lost moisture into the hair.

THE GRAYS

"Men look mature and need not worry too much about going gray. The gray/salt and pepper look is very distinguished on men and many carry this look well (think Richard Gere and Sean Connery!)" —Frédéric Fekkai

One of the most dramatic age-related changes that every man eventually experiences is graying hair. For the most part, the patterns and timing of the loss of pigment in the hair are genetically determined. Hair turns gray because of the lack of melanin pigment due to decreased melanocyte function, which is irreversible. Hair typically turns gray as a result of aging. Pigment in the hair shaft comes from special cells at the root (base) of the hair. These cells are genetically programmed to make a certain amount of pigment (melanin) at specific ages. At some point in the aging process, these cells make less and less pigment until the hair has very little pigment. White hair has no pigment, and gray hair has some but not as much as a red, black, or brown hair.

Not all hairs respond in the same way or at the same time. So the graying process usually is gradual. Graying cannot be prevented. Some men start graying in their 20s, and others do not see their first gray hair until their 60s. Men rarely go gray overnight. If they do, it is typically due to alopecia areata which causes the thicker, darker hairs to stop growing before it affects the growth of gray hairs giving the impression of graying overnight. Alopecia areata eventually causes patches of hair loss or complete loss of hair on the head or body.

If prematurely graying, look at the parents. Blondes, redheads, and light brunettes usually turn gray, whereas darker browns and blacks more commonly turn white. Fewer men today leave their hair gray or white, although some choose to keep it that way. As one ages, everything gets lighter as pigment fades, including the complexion. Gray hair can take on a yellowish tinge from the effects of sun, wind, and pollution. Try using shampoos and conditioners specially formulated to reduce the yellow tints. Extra conditioning is needed for gray or white hair, which tends to be more coarse and dry. As the cortex goes, the hair also tends to get more wiry, which can make it harder to manage.

To hide the gray, consider these chemical processes:

Permanent Color—Permanent color treats most heads, but it also the most potentially damaging. Two simple chemicals make all permanent colors work: hydrogen peroxide (sometimes called a developer or an activator) and ammonia. These swell the cuticle, remove at least a little natural pigment, and deposit the dye. Unfortunately, this process causes damage to the cuticle and destroys some of the protein in your hair. Ammonia can dry out the hair, cause frizz, and flatten out the color. Permanent color will last until the hair is cut or until it grows out, whichever comes first. Touch up the roots every four to six weeks.

Semi-Permanent Color—Gentler than permanent color, these liquid, gel, or foam formulas penetrate the hair shaft and stain the cuticle layer, but the color fades with every shampoo. No peroxide or ammonia is used. As it fades, the contrast between the ends and the roots will not be as noticeable. Because permanent and semi-permanent colors rough up the cuticle, hair can probably appear thicker after coloring. Semi-permanent color lasts six to eight weeks.

Temporary Color—These products deposit a translucent layer of dye on the outside of the cuticle and generally wash out after one or two shampoos. However, using them too often results in buildup. Temporary colors are a good way to experiment, to create interesting highlights, camouflage very small amounts of gray, or to freshen up fading permanent or semi-permanent coloring. Blue and purple rinses can be used to tone down yellowing in white hair and correct brassiness. Temporary color lasts one to two shampoos.

Color Preservation:

- Use only products with low alcohol content
- Wait at least 24 hours before washing hair after color
- Wash less frequently
- Avoid dry heat, chlorine, and direct sun exposure
- Use a UV protection conditioner or spray

SPLITTING HAIRS—HAIR LOSS UPDATE

As men age, the rate of hair growth slows. The most common cause of thinning hair is heredity and can be passed down from either the mother's or the father's side of the family. If suffering from excessive hair loss, before setting off on a search for hair transplants, the first step should be a consultation with a dermatologist to determine the cause. Some hair loss is temporary and will resolve without intervention. The condition of the hair reflects one's general health; it is a lagging indicator of your overall well being.

Diet Details

To prevent hair loss, pay attention to what is eaten because hair growth is related to diet. Temporary hair loss may result from the stress and shock that crash dieting puts on your internal systems. Deficiencies of protein or iron may impact hair count. The diet should have plenty of protein: meat, poultry, and foods that contain essential fatty acids, especially olive oil, and fish. Abnormal hair texture, sheen, and color can be a symptom of malnutrition. Supplemental vitamin pills, however, cannot prevent hair loss that is associated with rapid weight loss. Many over-the-counter diet supplements are high in vitamin A, which often makes hair loss worse.

- To keep hair healthy, get sufficient vitamins and minerals daily. A basic one-a-day vitamin supplement should be sufficient. It is important as well that the diet provide essential proteins, such as fish, meat, fowl, cheese, or simply three glasses of skim milk

- Though emotional and/or physical stress will not cause balding, these can adversely affect the quality and strength of the hair

- Try to protect the hair from harsh natural conditions, such as wind, cold weather, and sun, all of which tend to affect negatively the integrity of the hair

Good hair hygiene is essential to promote healthy hair. Always use a mild shampoo, as minimal an amount as possible, and only as often as necessary to keep it clean (for some men this will be once per day, others need to wash only every two to four days). Surroundings, including job, environment, and urban living can also be harsh on the hair. Conditioner should only be used for hair that is dry.

Thinning Hair

Areas of hair that no longer need cutting, and where the hairs are getting shorter and finer may be apparent. It is important to know that finding hairs in your tub, sink, or brush is not necessarily a sign of thinning hair. This could indicate a temporary hair loss condition. It is natural for hair to go through a constant cycle of growth and resting or dormancy. If not on the way to balding, the hair will grow back just as strong. If balding, the hair will grow back finer, and will not grow as long before falling out again. What is seen in the mirror over a longer period is the best monitor of early signs of thinning.

Hair loss can also be an indication of internal causes such as vitamin and mineral deficiencies, a low blood count, anemia, illness, hormonal changes, or the body's response to surgery or anesthesia. It can be a symptom of a variety of health-related factors, including thyroid abnormalities and autoimmune disease. Exposure to certain chemicals such as lithium salts, lead, mercury, selenium, arsenic, thallium, and borates can lead to hair loss. It can also be a result of taking some antibiotics, beta-blockers, antidepressants, and drugs for cholesterol and arthritis.

THE HAIR LOSS CONNECTION	
DRUGS LINKED TO HAIR LOSS	
Amphetamines, diet pills	Gout drugs
Antibiotics	Male hormones -
Anti-coagulants	Non Steroidal Anti-inflammatories (NSAIDs)
Anti-convulsants (Epilepsy)	Parkinsons Disease drugs
Anti-depressants	Radiation Agents (radio therapy)
Beta blockers (high blood pressure)	Thyroid drugs
Chemotherapy agents	Ulcer drugs
Cholesterol drugs	Vitamin A derivatives (Tretinoin)

TYPES OF HAIR LOSS

Androgenetic Alopecia

For men, this type of baldness is typically characterized by hair loss that begins at the temples and crown. The end result may be partial or complete baldness.

About 90 percent of the hair is in a two- to six-year growth (anagen) stage at any given time. The other 10 percent is in a two- to three-month resting (telogen) phase, after which time it is shed. Most people shed fifty to one hundred fifty hairs a day. Once a hair is shed, the growth stage begins again as a new hair from the same follicle replaces the shed hair. New hair grows at a rate of approximately one-half inch each month. Hair loss may lead to baldness when the rate of shedding exceeds the rate of regrowth, when new hair is thinner than the hair shed or when hair comes out in patches.

A history of androgenetic alopecia on either side of the family increases the risk of balding. Heredity also effects the age at which hair loss is begun and the developmental speed, pattern, and extent of baldness. Baldness, whether permanent or temporary, cannot be cured. There are treatments to help promote hair growth or hide hair loss. For some types of alopecia, hair may resume growth without any form of treatment.

Other Causes of Hair Loss

Anagen effluvium—generally results from medications administered internally, such as chemotherapy agents that poison the growing hair follicle.

Telogen effluvium—occurs because of an increased number of hair follicles entering the resting stage. When the causes are reversed or altered, you should see the return of normal hair growth. For example, if it is caused by certain medications you are taking, stopping the medication should reverse the hair loss. The most common causes are:

- Physical stress: surgery, illness, fever, infection, anemia, and rapid weight change
- Thyroid abnormalities
- Medications: high does of vitamin A, blood pressure medications, gout medications
- Hormonal changes

Emotional Stress

The body simply shuts down production of hair during periods of stress since it is not necessary for survival and instead devotes its energies toward repairing vital body structures. In many cases, there is a three-month delay between the actual event and the onset of hair loss. Furthermore, there may be another three-month delay before noticeable hair regrowth. Thus, the total hair loss and regrowth cycle can last six months or possibly longer when caused by physical or emotional stress. Though stress will not cause balding on its own, it can adversely affect the quality and strength of the hair. Stress also does not cause permanent hair loss.

"Some men look great bald, but for those who fear losing their hair, I recommend seeking the help of a hair treatment specialist. One tip I highly recommend is not to try and cover balding with a short-term solution (i.e. the comb over or a toupee). This usually brings more attention to the hair."—Frédéric Fekkai

Growth Stimulators

The effectiveness of medications used to treat hair loss depends on the cause of hair loss, the extent of the loss and individual response. Generally, treatment is less effective for more extensive cases of hair loss.

Minoxidil (Rogaine®)—Minoxidil is a liquid that is rubbed into the scalp twice daily to regrow hair and to prevent further loss. Some men experience hair regrowth or a slower rate of hair loss or both. Minoxidil is available in a 2 percent solution and in a 5 percent solution. New hair resulting from minoxidil use may be thinner and shorter than previous hair. But there can be enough regrowth for some people to hide their bald spots and have it blend with existing hair. New hair stops growing soon after you discontinue the use of minoxidil. Side effects can include irritation of the scalp.

Finasteride (Propecia®, Proscar®)—This prescription medication to treat male-pattern baldness is taken daily in pill form. Many people taking finasteride experience a slowing of hair loss, and some may show some new hair growth. Positive results may take several months. Finasteride works by inhibiting the conversion of testosterone into dihydrotestosterone (DHT), a hormone that shrinks hair follicles and is an important factor in male hair loss. Propecia® is very effective in slowing hair loss in the crown area, though it is less effective frontally. The short-term side-effects include decreased sex drive and erectile dysfunction which resolve as soon as use is discontinued. As with minoxidil, the benefits of finasteride stop if usage is discontinued.

Corticosteroids—Injections of cortisone into the scalp can treat alopecia areata. Treatment is usually repeated monthly. Corticosteroids may be prescribed for extensive hair loss due to alopecia areata. Ointments and creams can also be used, but they may be less effective than injections.

Anthralin (Drithocreme®)—Available as either a cream or an ointment, anthralin is a tarry substance applied to the scalp and washed off daily. Anthralin may stimulate new hair growth for cases of alopecia areata.

There are certain drugs that are used to treat hair loss that are considered 'off-label' uses, which means that they are not officially approved for hair loss although they may be approved for other conditions. Many drugs start out being prescribed for 'off-label' uses and eventually do get approved for the condition they are being used to treat after doctors and drug companies have collected enough clinical data.

Biotin is also indicated for healthy hair and skin, healthy sweat glands, nerve tissue, and bone marrow, and assisting in muscle pain. Biotin should be taken with the b-group vitamins, but vitamin C, vitamin B 5 (pantothenic acid), vitamin B 12, and sulfur are good companions to it.

TRANSPLANT TECHNIQUES

There is good news for men considering hair transplant surgery but who fear ending up with a corn row effect. Improved surgical techniques can achieve better hair follicle survival, take less time to perform, and leave fewer scars at the back and sides of the head. In one study, surgeons reported that the single-scar surgical technique for hair transplant surgery is a viable method that should be used more extensively. Although the single-scar technique is used by half of all hair transplant surgeons, it is not more common because it takes longer. A hair transplant surgeon should have extensive knowledge of the scalp anatomy at the ridge on the back of the head.

In most hair transplant procedures, healthy hair follicles are excised surgically from the back of the head where hair growth is permanent and thicker. Several methods overcome the obstacles that have deterred extensive use of the single-scar technique in place of multiple scars or a thick unsightly scar on the back of the head. An aesthetically pleasing, thin scar at the donor site after multiple hair-restoration procedures is the ultimate goal.

It is often counterproductive to use single hair follicles exclusively in hair transplant surgeries. In cases where follicular units are extremely close together, it is better to harvest them as three-or-four haired follicular groupings to assure better follicle survival rates. As a result, the multiple hair grafts are detached from the scalp for a shorter period of time, which increases the chances for successful transplantation. Transplanting groups of hair follicles can improve the cosmetic appeal of hair restoration and reduce excessively long procedures that were once common when transplanting single follicular units only.

MALE TALE: Eugene started losing his hair when he was in his early thirties. When it started happening, he thought it was the end of the world. He had a really hard time accepting the fact that he was going bald at such an early age. Although he knew about hair transplantation, he did not think he was a candidate because he was so young. Like many men, he had seen someone who had had a bad transplant so he did not pursue it. He tried hairpieces, which also looked awful, so one day his girlfriend told him to just forget about it. And he did, for at least a few years, but deep down he wished he could have at least enough hair to run a comb through. At 40, he came to see me about some liposuction on his lower belly. Eugene was a perfect candidate for liposuction, in great shape with just a slightly full abdomen. During his consultation, he brought up his hair thinning problem and asked me if anything could be done. I told him a friend of mine who had undergone one session of follicular unit hair transplants with a dermatologic surgeon. The results looked very natural and it cost around $8,000. Eugene ended up having his stomach liposuctioned in my surgical suite, and then he made an appointment for his hair. Eugene said, "Now that I have six-pack abs, I should have rock star hair to complete the look." The next time he came in for a checkup, he had a new head of hair. "Hey, I'll never be Bon Jovi, but at least there's something there now."

FLAKE RELIEF

Dandruff is actually a mild form of eczema, and it has many causes, including stress, sweating, and it can be present in dry or oily scalps. Although it can be quite unsightly, it is easily treated with antimicrobials or over the counter medicated shampoos that contain coal tar, salicylic acid (beta hydroxy acid), selenium sulfide, or zinc pyrithione. Dandruff shampoos can be drying, so use only as often as needed. Use a shampoo for dry hair and conditioner the rest of the time. Prescription strength sulfur, ketoconazole, and topical steroids may also be used to treat dandruff. In more severe forms of dandruff, the flakes are oilier and more yellowish than garden variety dandruff, and the scalp may be red and inflamed. This could be seborrheic dermatitis, which usually requires medical treatment.

Expert Tips

- Heavy conditioners and styling products designed to coat the hair can prevent the natural shedding of the scalp, hence a buildup of flakes
- Dry scalp is a common occurrence in winter from heating and lack of moisture in the air
- The scalp might be reacting to harsh ingredients in your shampoo. Switching to a gentler product may reduce flaking
- Clarifying shampoos that contain cider may reduce product build-up and lessen flakes
- Tea tree oil can be helpful as an antiseptic
- Get a scalp massage

SHAVING RITUALS

Choosing the right razor depends on two factors: first, skin type, and second, style. Electric razors work best on sensitive skin and for trimming beards. An electric razor can also give you a purposeful, rugged shag.

To keep from bleeding, take a shower before shaving to soften the skin, open up the pores, and reduce puffiness caused by sleep, all of which can cause nicks, cuts, and razor burn. If hurried, use a steamy washcloth and warm water instead. After showering, wash the face and neck with warm water and a mild cleanser to help remove the natural oils and perspiration that keep water from penetrating. Applying warm water causes hair to expand, making it softer and easier to cut. The force required to cut beard hair is reduced by almost 70 percent after two-minutes of warm water. Next, exfoliate with a special exfoliating cream or cleanser. This will get rid of dead skin around the hair so it can be cut closer to the root. As a result, the shave will be smoother and last longer.

After washing the face, it is time to apply shaving cream. For the best results, use a shave brush made with badger hair not synthetic bristles. Badger hair bristles retain water really well, which when mixed with shaving cream provides an effective barrier, preventing the blade from dragging and skipping across the skin. A brush made from badger hair bristles will also last longer than one made with synthetic bristles because badger hair is pliant and remains soft. Technique: treat the shave brush like a paintbrush: the face is the canvas so apply gently and stroke sideways otherwise the bristles will break if the brush is pressed onto the skin. Let your brush dry in the open air. Apply plenty of shaving cream or gel. Although water is the essential softening agent, the water absorbed by hair quickly evaporates, leaving the hair in its original rigid state. Shaving cream or gel provides a protective blanket that prevents the evaporation of water and keeps beard hair soft during the shave. Additionally, the lubricating characteristics of shaving cream and gel reduce friction between blade and skin, improving razor glide for a smoother shaving experience. Choose a shave gel designed specifically for the skin type.

Always remember to use sharp a blade. A crusted, rusted blade may cut the skin instead of the hair. Remember not to hurry, use short strokes and a light touch, going with the growth of the hair, which varies from spot to spot—usually sideways under the chin and down on the cheeks. Start with the side burns, then move to your cheeks, neck, and finish with upper lip and chin—the whiskers are coarse here so the extra time will allow the cream to soften them up. While shaving, frequently dip the razor in hot water to clear out hairs and excess cream and to keep the blade sharp. The life of a blade is one week; four or five days if you have a beard. Leave hard-to-shave spots for last; shave cheeks, sides of face, and neck first. Occasionally, a second attempt will shave even closer. This time shave against the direction of hair growth.

Rinse the face and neck with cool water and pat dry; do not rub. To prevent stinging and irritation, use a non-alcohol based aftershave, preferably one that also moisturizes to keep the skin soft. When selecting an aftershave, pay attention to your skin type. A product made for one's skin type makes a big difference: your skin will be smooth, not greasy. At the end of every shave, rinse the blade thoroughly and shake off excess water before storing. Do not wipe the blade as this can damage the fine shaving edge.

GETTING A CLOSE SHAVE

- Take a hot shower to open up your pores

- Dry your face and neck with a soft towel

- Apply and massage in a small amount of shaving oil to all areas of the face and neck where planned to shave

- Run a shaving brush under hot water and lather up either a shaving cream or soap to create a rich lather

- Begin shaving in the direction of the grain (the direction of hair growth). Do not push down to hard on the razor because it will cause you to have razor burns

- Re-lather the face and neck area with a light lather and shave very lightly against or adjacent to the grain

- Wash the face with cold water to remove excess shaving cream/soap which was not used

- Run the tip of an alum block under cold water until the stone is moistened. Apply the alum block to all areas of the face and neck where shaved for it will act as an antiseptic

- Apply a small amount of after shave balm or gel to the areas of the face where just shaved

Soy-infused shaving creams can slow the growth of facial hair and make the stubble on the neck less coarse. In addition, soy appears to help eliminate bumps and ingrown hairs.

Shaving Factoids

- Age at which the average adolescent began shaving: 14
- Number of times the average guy shaves each week: 5

Solving Shaving Bumps

Occurring in the beard area, pseudo-folliculitis barbae (PFB), commonly known as shaving bumps, is a widespread problem among men with curly hair and dark skin. As the hair follicle grows out of the skin, it immediately curls and re-enters the skin. The skin reacts to it as a foreign body and becomes inflamed, swollen, and irritated, thereby creating bumps. Blade shaving exacerbates the problem by sharpening ends of the hairs like a spear. Over time, this can cause keloidal scarring which looks like hard bumps of the beard area and neck. Sometimes these bumps become quite large.

The most effective treatment is to let the beard grow. Once the hairs get to be a certain length, they will not grow back into the skin. Washing the beard area with an exfoliant raises the hairs from under the skin and prevents them from growing back into the skin. This should be done twice a day.

Solving Shaving Bumps

- Use an electric razor because it does not cut as close as blades do

- Shave every other day, rather than daily

- Do not pull the skin taut when blade shaving

- Avoid using a double or triple-edged razor

- If a blade must be used, before shaving, wash the face with a mild cleanser, then rinse

- Massage the beard area gently in a circular motion with a warm, moist, soft washcloth to free up the hair tips so they can be cut with the shaver. Use warm water to soften the hairs, making them easier to cut

- Lather the beard area with a non-irritating shaving gel instead of cream and shave in the direction of beard growth

- After shaving, rinse thoroughly with warm water and apply a mild moisturizing aftershave lotion

- Do not pull the in-grown hair out which can cause infection and scarring

Bumps can also be somewhat relieved by using topical steroids, retinoids such as Retin-A®, or a topical antibiotic solution prescribed by a doctor can help the problem. Other options include laser treatments to remove the hair follicles. Medications are also prescribed to speed healing of the skin. Glycolic acid lotion, prescription antibiotic gels (Benzamycin, Cleocin-T), or oral antibiotics are also effective. Retin-A® is a potent treatment that helps even out any scarring after a few months. It is added as a nightly application of Retin-A® Cream 0.05 - 0.1% to the beard skin while beard is growing out. Use as tolerated, as it may be irritating.

GROOM & TRIM—MUSTACHE, BEARDS, NOSE

Unfortunately as one ages, ears get bigger and grow some hair, glasses get thicker, and nose hairs get longer. Nose hairs can easily be taken care of in the privacy of one's own home with a good trimmer.

HAIR REMOVAL

Along with wrinkles and sagging skin, aging is also marked by an increase of hair on the brow, ears, back, and chest. With a little prompting, most men are adept at the basics of dressing right, smelling great, and making sure that every strand on their heads is in place, but they sometimes overlook the hair on their back. Today, the image of masculinity portrayed in magazines is of a well-built man with a smooth chest and back.

BODY HAIR

The amount of body, facial, and scalp hair can vary significantly over one's lifetime. Genetics are the main determinate of a hair pattern and the amount of hair you have.

Male hormones (androgens) influence hair growth on some areas of the body while other areas respond very little. Androgen-dependent areas of body hair include the pubic area, armpits, face, chest, abdomen, and scalp. Some parts of the scalp may respond to androgen stimulation with hair loss while other areas respond with hair growth.

The finer hairs on the arms and legs are less dependent on hormones.

The degree to which an androgen-dependent area responds to hormonal changes is also genetically determined. For example, one man may have a large amount of hair on his chest and abdomen while another may have very little. Hormone levels are no higher, but the skin is genetically programmed to respond by growing hair.

Male hormone levels rise as adrenal glands and testicles mature. Often this results in hair growth in the pubic and armpit areas and, with individual variation, hair growth on the face and body, and hair loss on the scalp.

These changes can continue through adulthood. It is not uncommon to continue to develop a thick beard or more body hair through the thirties, forties and fifties. Similarly, scalp hair loss can begin in the teens and progress at varying rates through adulthood. Baldness typically begins with a regression of the hairline at the forehead and thinning at the crown of your head.

A significant decline in body, armpit, and pubic hair—especially if associated with other signs and symptoms such as decreased libido, erectile dysfunction, fatigue, lightheadedness, breast enlargement or tenderness, or weight changes—may indicate a hormonal problem requiring a doctor's evaluation. But if scalp hair is lost in patches, see a dermatologist.

Grooming Preferences

Almost all women dislike hair on the back, but are too embarrassed to tell their mate. According to a Harris Interactive survey of 1,000, more than 90 percent of women between the ages of eighteen and forty-four find back hair to be unattractive. Yet, despite their aversion to back hair, only four in ten women would ever feel comfortable asking their significant other to handle their hairy hang-up. Though one in three men currently removes hair from unwanted areas of their bodies, including their back, chest, and legs, survey results indicate that women are looking for more men to incorporate hair removal into their normal grooming routine. When asked in confidence, the women surveyed ranked the back as the number one area of their man's body they desired to see smooth (77 percent). The derriere ranked second with 11 percent of women desiring a buff butt followed by the chest at seven percent. Not surprisingly, most women did not mind a little hair on arms and legs.

Permanent Hair Removal

Innovative, light-based devices have revolutionized the treatment of unwanted hair, offering gentle, effective, and convenient solutions for men. Most systems use targeted flashes of light to block the re-growth potential of the hair follicle. One may be more suitable than the other, based on the patient's skin-type. The light-based energy actually damages or destroys hair follicles at the cellular level. These treatments do not damage surrounding tissue and each device targets numerous hair follicles simultaneously, allowing for the treatment of large areas quickly and effectively. A permanent reduction in the number of hairs that grow back is usually achieved following each treatment. This technology can be used to treat unwanted hair on all skin types, including dark-skinned individuals such as those of African, Hispanic, or Asian descent, as well as those patients with tanned skin. Any hair with at least some pigment can be treated.

The length of a single treatment may last anywhere from a few minutes to an hour or more, depending on the size of the area being treated. The number of treatments required depends on several factors related to thickness and density of hair and types and color of skin. It is important to understand that hairs in an active growth phase (anagen) are most affected by treatments. Since all hairs are not in this phase at the same time, several treatments are necessary to achieve the best results. Subsequent sessions are scheduled when the hair begins to regrow. The timing for this can range from four to eight weeks, depending on hair type and the part of the body being treated. A customized treatment program is designed, so the number of sessions varies from man to man. On average, treatments are scheduled four to six weeks apart.

Before each session begins, system settings are computer-customized according to skin color and type and the area of the body being treated. Treatment begins by trimming away any hair above the surface of the skin and then conducting test spots to determine the patient's skin response to different device settings. Next, a cold gel (similar to ultrasound gel) is spread over the treatment area. This helps keep the skin cool and focus the light treatment. The handpiece is moved over the treatment area, while light-based energy is emitted in highly controlled flashes or pulses. This heats up the hair, significantly damaging the regrowth potential of the follicle. When the gel is removed, much of the hair is wiped off with it. Additional hair may fall out over the next week or two.

The treatment may cause some minor discomfort or a slight tingling, often compared to a pinch or the sting of a snapped rubber band. Most patients tolerate the procedure well. Topical anesthesia can be used when treating particularly sensitive areas of the body.

The appearance of the treated area immediately following a session will vary from patient to patient, though side effects are rare. Any swelling or redness at the treatment site typically goes away within a couple of hours, and most men are able to return to normal activity immediately. Many of the unwanted hairs are gone at the end of the treatment. The appearance of the treated area immediately following treatment will vary from patient to patient depending on the extent of the procedure and skin type. On rare occasions, some blistering may occur, but this typically resolves quickly. The skin can become darker or lighter following treatment, but will generally return to normal within a few weeks. Limiting sun exposure before and after each treatment will minimize the risk of complications.

Intense Pulsed Light (IPL) Systems for Hair Removal

The IPL system uses broadband of light spectrum to damage hair follicles for long-term hair removal. Each system has shown to be a successful method for reducing unwanted, unsightly hairs. Unlike conventional laser systems, the wavelengths of the IPL system emit light energy in very carefully timed bursts to:

- Maximize the effectiveness of the treatment

- Decrease the potential for injury to the surrounding skin

- Minimize discomfort

IPL systems treat the hair by directing light energy through a light guide placed on the patient's skin. A thin layer of transparent gel covers the treatment area to focus the light energy and cool the top skin layer. The light energy heats and damages the hair follicle, typically causing the hair itself to fall out from the follicle. The IPL system is gentle, non-invasive, and has minimal side effects.

IPL system treatment parameters can be selected according to an individual's specific skin color, hair color, and hair density. This allows customization of each individual treatment based on personal experience, as well as the unique attributes of the hair follicles. As a result of this computer-generated precision, the IPL system is effective on a wide range of hair colors, from blonde through auburn to brown and dark black hair. The IPL system successfully removes hair from all skin types, even dark brown complexions, and from any part of the body, no matter how deep the follicles may reside. Treatment of sensitive areas such as the ears, nose, and underarms can be tolerated with minimal discomfort. Another advantage is its wide treatment area, enabling the device to treat patients rapidly. In fact, approximately one- to two-hundred hairs can be treated with each flash of the light, so that large areas on the back and chest can be treated in a single session. Multiple treatment sessions of four to six are typically required for long-lasting hair removal.

LASER HAIR REDUCTION

The laser beam or a light pulse works to destroy the hair bulb itself. Multiple sessions may be required, but it can be used on many parts of the body where unwanted hair may appear.

Melanin-Targeting Lasers

Ruby, alexandrite, and flashlamp are the three types of energy that are effective upon melanin in hair. All supply a wavelength of light that is absorbed by melanin. They are most effective on light-skinned men with dark hair. If used on men with dark skin, normal skin pigment may be damaged. The primary drawback with these lasers is the lack of effectiveness on very light or white hairs and the limitations of treating tanned or dark skin.

Ruby Lasers

A number of available systems utilize ruby lasers with various methods of delivery. Although these systems are designed to deliver maximum light energy to the follicle with minimum impact on the epidermal skin, there are potential risks of short-term loss of skin color (hypopigmentation) and blistering. Men with light skin and dark hair have the best outcomes. Men with light-colored hair are not good candidates for this laser.

Alexandrite Lasers

In addition to melanin, these lasers also allow absorption by hemoglobin (a red pigment in the red blood cells). One system has the capability to deliver rapid pulses with lengths as short as twenty milliseconds, offering the potential for a more focused hair reaction with decreased injury to the skin.

Flashlamp Lasers

This system applies a broad band of energy directed to the tissue, generated by a flashlamp rather than a single wavelength of a laser.

Nd:YAG

The Nd:YAG utilizes a carbon-based cream to loosen hair from the follicle and was the first type of laser to be FDA-approved for hair removal.

Treatment Areas

The back, shoulders, arms, and legs are areas typically treated with laser light. Certain areas such as the shoulder (deltoid region) and chest (presternal region) should be avoided due to the increased risk of scarring and keloid formation.

What Are the risks?

Localized trauma such as blistering after treatment and short-term hypo- or hyperpigmentation, which usually resolves, may occur. Other rare risks include scarring, keloid formation, and infection (viral, fungal, or bacterial). Technologic advances ultimately will allow for more uniform application of light energy and more success in treating a wider range of men with dark skin and/or light hair.

TAMING THE BROWS

Slanted tweezers are ideal because an angle is needed to pull a hair out by the root. Tweezing is great to get at ingrown hairs, but it is also the best way to keep eyebrows in tip-top shape. The brow keeps sweat out of the eyes (eyelashes protect our eyes from dust). If a uni-brow (one long eye brow and not two) is present, a professional can shape up the brows to look best and remove any unruly, stray hairs. Since tweezing pulls the hair out by the root, it will take at least a week, maybe more or less depending on how fast the hair grows, before a hair will come back and will need to be tweezed again.

GROOMING ON THE GO: A DAILY ROUTINE

Cleanse—Wash the skin once a day (either by bath or shower) and use a cleanser for specific skin type. Keep showers short and your water tepid. Too much hot water depletes the body's moisture balance. When washing, avoid common alkaline soaps, which can dry the skin. Instead use nonalcohol shower gels, liquid cleansers, or nonsoap bars that are gentler on the skin. For oily skin, use a cleanser with alcohol to dissolve the oil. For dry skin, avoid products with alcohol or astringents because these products zap moisture.

Moisturize—Use a light gel or lotion moisturizer with an SPF 15 to protect skin. Apply the moisturizer while the face is still wet to seal in the moisture and draw water from the deeper layers of the skin. If skin is oily, only use moisturizers that are oil-free and non-comedogenic, to avoid clogging pores and causing breakouts. Oily, acne prone skin may only require the use of a light moisturizing formula only every other day.

Exfoliate—The body is covered with a nasty layer of dead skin. From the neck up, use a mild facial scrub to get rid of the dead skin. Do not apply too much pressure to avoid causing irritation. When removing dead skin cells off the surface, this will stimulate the skin to produce new cells and gives skin a smoother texture and healthy glow.

Shave—The best time to shave is when the bathroom is still steamed up, which helps soften the beard and make it easier to cut. Before shaving, apply a preshave oil to protect the skin, soften the beard, and help the razor glide evenly. Dark hair and a heavy beard increase the chances of razor burn and ingrown hairs. Then lather up with shaving cream. First shave with the grain, then go against the grain for the closest shave. This helps get rid of ingrown hairs, and it will leave the face feeling smooth. Use a three-blade razor for a faster shave. Follow with an aftershave balm instead of aftershave:

Comb—Use only the amount of product that you need, and do not overdo it. For fine hair, try a light mist of hair spray on damp hair. Lightly blow-dry for texture and volume. Next, apply a finishing cream to create a natural, thicker appearance. Avoid gels that turn brittle. For curly or frizzy hair, comb in a leave-in conditioner and some styling paste to smooth the hair and make it more manageable.

Pluck—The older a man, the more stray hairs he grows. Use a magnifying mirror to see tweeze, cut, or buzz stray hairs with a trimmer. Use a pair of small scissors to trim unruly brows.

Hands—Clean the fingernails and file them to trim. Buy a simple, functional nail-care kit. Soak the hands in water for a minute, then clean the nails, trim them, and push the cuticles back with a cuticle pusher. Trim the toenails, too.

Treatment—To decrease oil and acne, reduce the appearance of fine lines, wrinkles, and age spots, apply a topical retinoid before bed. Using a retinoid daily also may protect against skin cancers because it encourages cell turnover and eliminates precancerous, sun-damaged cells. Retinoids may cause flaking and redness, so be sure to use a moisturizer with sunscreen to keep the skin hydrated and to protect it from the increased sensitivity.

Care for Healthy, Comfortable Feet:

- Do not ignore foot pain—it is not normal. If pain persists, see a podiatrist
- Inspect feet regularly. Pay attention to changes in color and temperature. Look for thick or discolored nails (a sign of possible fungus), and check for cracks or cuts in the skin. Peeling or scaling on the soles of feet may indicate athlete's foot. Any growth on the foot is not considered normal
- Wash feet daily, especially between the toes, and be sure to rinse off all soap and dry them completely
- Trim toenails straight across, but not too short. Be careful not to cut nails in corners or on the sides; it can lead to ingrown toenails. Men with diabetes, poor circulation, or heart problems should not treat their own feet because they are more prone to infection
- Make sure that shoes fit properly. Purchase new shoes later in the day when feet tend to be at their largest and replace worn out shoes as soon as possible
- Select and wear the right shoe for each activity that you are doing
- Alternate shoes—do not wear the same pair of shoes every day
- Wear clean socks, changed daily. Do not wear socks that are too short or too tight
- Avoid walking barefoot—feet will be more prone to injury and infection. At the beach or when wearing sandals always use sun block on your feet as well as the rest of your body

Some men's feet sweat more than others and are more prone to athlete's foot.

- Wear shoes made of leather or canvas, not synthetics; sandals are good in warm, humid weather
- Switch your shoes daily
- Use foot powder in the shoes every day

ATHLETE'S FOOT

Athlete's foot (tinea pedis) is a common, persistent infection of the foot caused by a dermatophyte, a microscopic fungus that lives on dead tissue of the hair, toenails, and outer skin layers. These fungi thrive in warm, moist environments such as shoes, stockings, and the floors of public showers, locker rooms, and swimming pools.

Athlete's foot is transmitted through contact with a cut or abrasion on the bottom of the foot. In rare cases, the fungus is transmitted from infected animals to humans. Skin infections cause raised, circular pimples or blisters that resemble lesions caused by ringworm. Athlete's foot is most common in men from their teens to their early fifties, mostly because of their personal hygiene and daily activity. Common symptoms include persistent itching of the skin on the sole of the foot or between the toes, cracked skin, rashes, and bumps.

Antifungal drugs may be used to fight the infection. Clotrimazole (sold over-the-counter as Lotrimin) and miconazole (contained in Lotrimin and Absorbine Jr.), are available in cream, powder, spray, or liquid form and can be applied topically and massaged into the skin. Side effects are rare and include mild gastrointestinal distress and liver/kidney enzyme problems. Another imidazole drug, itraconazole (Sporanox) is available in capsule form. Other preparations in this class include Desenex and Tinactin, which contain tolnaftate. If the infection is bacterial, oral antibiotics may be prescribed.

NAIL IT

The basic tools are toenail clipper, fingernail clipper, and emery board to shape and reduce the size of the nails. Toenail clippers have a straight blade while the blade of fingernail clippers is curved. If fingernail clippers are used on the toes, then the nail will not grow to the shape of the toe and vice versa. The basic motion with the emery board is to start from the center of the nail and go on to the sides.

Ingrown Nails

Ingrown toenails are caused by the penetration of the edges of the nail plate into the soft tissue of the toe. It begins with a painful irritation that often becomes infected. With bacterial invasion, the nail margin becomes red and swollen, often showing drainage or pus. In men who have diabetes or poor circulation this seemingly minor problem can be become quite severe. Severe ingrown toenails can result in gangrene of the toe. There are several causes of ingrown toenails: a hereditary tendency to form ingrown toenails, improperly cutting the toenails either too short or cutting into the side of the nail, and ill-fitting shoes. Once an ingrown toenail starts, they will often recur. Many men cut the nail margin out only to have it recur months later as the nail grows out.

What Can Be Done?

Treatment for ingrown toenails involves removing the nail margin, which destroys the nail root in this area. Most commonly an acid will be used to kill the root of the nail. It may take a few weeks for the nail margin to heal completely, but there are generally no restrictions in activity, bathing, or wearing shoes. Recurrence of the ingrown toenail can occur. Continuation of the infection is possible, which can be controlled easily with oral antibiotics. On occasion, the remaining nail may become loose from the nail bed and fall off. The new nail will grow out to replace it over several months.

CORNS & CALLUSES

Corns and calluses are areas of thick skin that result form excessive pressure or friction over a boney prominence. When these areas develop on the top of the toes, they are called corns. When they occur on the bottom of the foot they are called calluses. They can also occur between the toes, the back of the heels, and the top of the foot. The thickening of the skin is a normal body response to pressure or friction. Often they are associated with a projection of bone called a bone spur. However, not all areas of thickened skin are corns or calluses. For example, plantar warts also cause a discreet thickening of the skin that resemble corns and calluses.

Corns

Corns are areas of thick skin that most commonly occur on the top of the toes. Generally there is an associated hammertoe deformity, which causes the toes to rub on the top of the shoes. Professional treatment is directed at correcting the hammertoe deformity. Small corns can also occur on the side of the little toe next to the toenail. A small bone spur causes this problem. Treatment consists of removing the bone spur. Bone spurs also cause corns between the toes. Soft corns are areas of white moist skin between the toes. They most commonly occur between the fourth and fifth toes. They can be very painful and if not treated can form small ulcerations that can become infected. A soft corn is due to an irregularity in the shape of the bone in the fourth or fifth toes.

What Can Be Done?

Home treatment should reduce the pressure between the toes with cotton or a foam cushion and using an antibiotic ointment to reduce the risk of infection. Treatment consists of removing the irregular shaped bone that causes the development of the corn. Some men prefer simply to trim down and to pad the calloused areas.

Calluses

The most common area for the formation of calluses on the bottom of the foot is on the ball of the foot. This is a weight bearing area where the long bones behind the toes bear the greatest amount of weight and pressure. If one or more of these long bones is out of alignment then excessive pressure is generated in the area and a callous forms. The callused area can be very discreet and have a "core" or they can be more dispersed covering a larger area. These areas can become quite painful as the skin thickens.

What Can Be Done?

There are numerous over the counter treatments for calluses. Some of these remedies have an acid in them that burn the callous off. These remedies are only temporary because the source of the pressure has not been alleviated. Professional treatment consists of using a special shoe insert called a functional orthotic that corrects foot function. In certain instances surgery may be recommended to correct the alignment of the offending bone. Cutting out the callous will only make the condition worse if the underling boney problem is not corrected. Metatarsal surgery may also be recommended if the problem persists.

SWEAT CONTROL

Hyperhidrosis, or excessive sweating, can be localized to one area or it may be generalized. In the localized type, the most common sites are the palms and soles of the feet. The cause of the excessive sweating is not well understood. There is an emotional component to it in some but not all cases. The excessive moisture contributes to athlete's foot and plantar wart infections.

BOTOX® FOR EXCESSIVE SWEATING

Hyperhidrosis is a rare condition in which large quantities of water and electrolytes are exuded from the body. In severe cases, the hands and feet may drip with secretions. The condition has a considerable emotional and social burden. When other treatments have failed, surgical intervention is possible, but the risk of compensatory sweating in other areas exists.

Botulinum toxin A is commercially manufactured as Botox®. Using botulinum toxin to inhibit sweat production is very effective. Treating armpit, hand, facial, and gustatory (related to salivation or eating) hyperhidrosis with botulinum toxin can last six months or longer in most cases.

LEG VEINS

While arteries carry blood away from the heart, veins carry blood to the heart. As the blood flows back to the heart, veins regulate blood flow, preventing the blood from flowing in the wrong direction. In some cases, especially over time, a vein may weaken, and some blood may trickle back into the vein. As the blood collects in the vein, it can become congested or clogged, causing the vein to swell. Dark, purple veins that rise above the skin's surface, called varicose veins, are quite large and swollen, and look unsightly, causing many to seek treatment. Varicose veins in men frequently appear on the backs of calves or on the inside of the leg, anywhere from the groin to the ankle.

Chart: Varicose Vein Triggers

- Heredity
- Excess sun exposure
- Weight gain
- Certain medications
- Prolonged standing
- Traumatizing the skin

VEIN TREATMENTS

Varicose vein treatment initially begins with attempts to compress the region with stockings or support hosiery. Graduated support stockings, which gently and evenly reduce fatigue, pain, and swelling, can help men suffering from poor circulation, edema, chronic venous insufficiency, and varicose veins. Wearing graduated support hosiery is the first step of varicose vein treatment. If wearing support stockings does not alleviate symptoms, other treatment options, including injections, laser skin surgery, or surgery to destroy the damaged veins, can be attempted. Another option is to pass a thin laser fiber into the vein that then releases a quick burst of laser light. The heat seals the vein and causes it to close and eventually disappear.

Even with treatment, however, the veins can return in other places on the body, so it is best to take preventative measures to avoid getting varicose veins in the first place. Protect the skin from the sun by avoiding exposure or wearing sunscreen when outside.

Avoiding Unsightly Veins

- Exercise to improve the strength of the veins and leg muscles

- Do not cross the legs

- Avoid wearing clothing that restricts circulation.

- Keep weight stable

- Standing for long periods of time can contribute to the likelihood of getting varicose veins

- Eat enough fiber; constipation can contribute to varicose veins

- Wear elastic support stockings on long flights to improve circulation

CHAPTER 11

Smile Rejuvenation

"Most men are actually unhappy with their teeth, but only a small percentage of men realize how incredibly simple it is to change their smiles. A smile makeover usually takes two visits that last a few hours each—it's that easy. People will notice you look great, but they won't know why."

—Marc Lowenberg, DDS,
New York City Cosmetic Dentist

No one can overestimate the importance of a great smile. A fresh new smile can disarm everyone you come in contact with, and it is one of the first things people notice. When uncomfortable with the way the teeth look, it can easily be misinterpreted in the smile. If you are embarrassed by your teeth, you have probably trained yourself subconsciously to hide them. Do you talk with your lips tightly pursed? Do you smile without actually opening up your lips? Do you ever place your hand over your smile when you laugh? These are some of the telltale signs that you are feeling self-conscious about your smile.

Many men are satisfied with the sparkle they get from brushing twice daily with a fluoride-containing toothpaste, cleaning between their teeth once a day, and regular professional cleanings. If one decides to go beyond this to make your smile look brighter, there are many options:

- Whitening toothpastes
- At-home bleaching
- In-office bleaching

Teeth whitening has become as commonplace as Botox® injections. Some teeth just start out dark while others become stained over time from smoking or drinking dark liquids. Some medications, such as the antibiotic tetracycline, can also darken teeth. If discolored teeth are visible, but are otherwise happy, bleaching may an option. Even a perfect smile will deteriorate as one ages. As one ages, the outer layer of enamel on the teeth wears away. Eventually it reveals the darker tissue underneath, at the center of the tooth around the nerves and blood vessels.

Whiteners may not correct all types of discoloration. For example, yellow-ish hued teeth will probably bleach well, brownish-colored teeth may bleach less well, and grayish-hued teeth may not bleach well at all. Likewise, bleaching may not enhance the smile if bonding or tooth-colored fillings have been placed in the front teeth. The whitener will not affect the color of these materials, and they will stand out in the newly whitened smile. In these cases, other options, such as porcelain veneers or dental bonding should be investigated.

If a candidate for bleaching, a dentist may suggest a procedure that can be done in his or her office. This procedure is called chairside bleaching and often requires multiple office visits. The dentist will apply either a protective gel to the gums or a rubber shield to protect the oral soft tissues. A bleaching agent is then applied to the teeth, and a special light may be used to enhance the action of the agent. Lasers have been used during tooth whitening procedures to enhance the action of the whitening agent.

Bleaching usually requires three to ten treatments, lasting about thirty minutes to an hour and a half. It is suggested that three or more professional cleaning be performed per year after treatments are completed to help keep teeth stain-free. Thorough brushing after meals is necessary to avoid plaque accumulation. Smoking and stain-causing foods such as coffee and tea should be avoided. Yellow and brown stains can be considerably reduced, though teeth may not be returned to natural color. Annual touch-ups may be required.

"While laser bleaching will not necessary look better than home bleaching, it will get you the desired result faster. The problem with any kind of bleaching, however, is that it is unpredictable and you do not always get an even or long-lasting result."—Marc Lowenberg, DDS

There are several types of products available for use at home, which can either be dispensed by your dentist or purchased over-the-counter.

Bleaching Solutions—These products contain peroxide(s), which actually bleach the tooth enamel. These products typically rely on carbamide peroxide as the bleaching agent. Carbamide peroxide comes in several different concentrations (10, 16, and 22 percent). Peroxide-containing whiteners typically come in a gel and are placed in a mouthguard. Usage regimens vary. Some products are used twice a day for two weeks, and others are intended for overnight use for one to two weeks. A dentist can make a custom-fitted mouthguard that will fit the teeth precisely. Teeth can become sensitive during the period when using the bleaching solution. In many cases, this sensitivity is temporary and should lessen once the treatment is finished. Some men also have soft tissue irritation—either from a tray that does not fit properly or from solution that may come in contact with the tissues.

Toothpastes—All toothpastes help remove surface stains through the action of mild abrasives. Whitening toothpastes usually contain chemical or polishing agents that provide additional stain removal effectiveness, however, the results are variable and not dramatic from whitening toothpastes alone.

PORCELAIN LAMINATES

"Porcelain veneers can totally transform your smile. We are able to contour the teeth to match the face, rather than just installing the identical "Hollywood" white smile for every man. The newly developed porcelain laminates are more translucent and offer the kind of natural-looking correction that men really want."—Marc Lowenberg, DDS

There is no reason to put up with gaps in the teeth or with teeth that are stained, badly shaped, or crooked. The best cosmetic dentistry requires a highly personalized approach and good communication between the patient and the dentist. There is no substitute for a critical aesthetic eye and years of experience.

Bleaching is temporary, and may last one to two years, whereas porcelain veneers can transform a smile and last ten to twenty years. Most people looking for a movie-star smile are mainly interested in whitening, at least for starters. Today a porcelain laminate placed on top of the teeth can correct nature's mistakes or the results of an injury and help create a beautiful smile. Veneers are thin, custom-made shells crafted of tooth-colored materials designed to cover the front side of teeth. They are made by a dental technician, usually in a dental lab, working from a model provided by a dentist. With porcelain veneers, virtually anything can be done to improve a smile. They are like little shells that wrap around the tooth to create different shapes and varying shades for a totally flawless yet natural look.

Laminates usually require two office visits. The teeth will be prepared and an impression made during the first visit, which can take one to four hours. The laminates will be fitted and inserted at the second visit, which may also take the same amount of time.

"Not only can porcelain veneers give you the perfect color and brightness, but we can also change the shape of your teeth, close spaces, fix chips, straighten teeth that are crooked—it is like instant orthodontics. The added benefit is that porcelain doesn't stain, so you can drink coffee, tea and red wine without any worries."—Marc Lowenberg, DDS

The teeth should be professionally cleaned three to four times yearly. Warn the hygienist not to use ultrasonic scaling or air abrasive. Also take precautions with eating habits. As with bonding and crowning, take special care when biting into or chewing hard foods with laminated teeth because laminates are not as strong as enamel. Margins eventually need resealing. The effect is a polished, natural-appearing result that effectively masks stains. Laminates can last fifteen years if cared for properly.

CROWNING

For a smile that is the crowning glory, a crown may be needed to cover a tooth and restore it to its normal shape and size. A crown can make a tooth stronger and improve its appearance. It can cover and support a tooth with a large filling when there is not enough tooth left. It can be used to attach a bridge, protect a weak tooth from breaking, or restore one that is already broken. A crown is a good way to cover teeth that are discolored or badly shaped. It is also used to cover a dental implant. Crowns usually require two appointments of approximately one to four hours each for up to four teeth. Expect to spend more time as additional teeth or more extensive treatments are involved. Crowns are designed to look and feel like real teeth.

Tooth fractures such as biting down on hard things like peanut brittle or ice must be avoided. A decay-free diet that reduces the intake of refined sugars is imperative to prevent the cement that holds the crowns in place from washing away. Have a professional cleaning at least three or four times yearly. Fluoride treatments should be given once a year. Flossing at least once per day is essential for crowns. The most beautiful results with full crowns can be destroyed if the teeth decay beneath the crowns.

Crowning can achieve the ultimate in shade control, tooth shape, and size. The average aesthetic life of the full crown is five to fifteen years. Life expectancy is directly proportional to three things: fracture, problems with tissue, and the hidden danger of decay.

ORTHODONTICS

Orthodontics requires six to thirty-six months for most adults and special care by cleaning daily and check ups on a scheduled basis. Retainers frequently have to be worn at night for many years, at least a few nights a week, possibly indefinitely, to maintain tooth alignment. A water-powered cleaning device is also helpful if used daily. With orthodontics, spaces between teeth are closed, and the results are generally permanent.

INVISALIGN®

As an alternative to traditional orthodontia, Invisalign® uses a series of clear plastic, removable aligners to straighten teeth gradually, without metal or wires. The plastic trays, which are custom-made and resemble teeth-whitening trays, work by moving the teeth incrementally. Each tray is worn all day (except when eating or brushing) for about two weeks, then the next tray in the series is used until the final position is achieved. Like brackets and archwires, these aligners move teeth through the controlled force. At each stage, only designated teeth move in order to maximize efficiency.

The Invisalign® system is nearly invisible, removable, and comfortable. Teeth can be straightened without the appearance or hassle of braces, including a restricted diet and trouble flossing or brushing. However, with Invisalign, smoking or chewing gum is prohibited. Smoking can discolor the trays, while gum will stick to them. Temporary, minor discomfort is to be expected for a few days at the beginning of each new stage of treatment. This is normal and a sign that treatment is working to move the teeth. Besides pain, the aligners affect speech, but as the tongue adjusts, any lisp or speech impediment should disappear. Aligners need to be cleaned daily with lukewarm water. During treatment, regular appointments—usually about once every six weeks—will be scheduled with the orthodontist to make sure that treatment is progressing correctly.

COSMETIC CONTOURING

Contouring or tooth reshaping is used either to correct crooked, chipped, cracked, or overlapping teeth or to alter the length, shape, or position of the teeth in just one to three office visits. In some cases, this technique is substituted for braces. The changes, although subtle, may produce enough cosmetic improvement to enhance the overall appearance of the smile. Only a few millimeters of reduction can create a beautiful smile. Teeth may become weaker if large amounts of enamel are removed. Therefore, tooth reshaping is generally limited to minor changes or combined with veneers for best results.

A sanding drill or laser may be used to remove small amounts of surface enamel gradually. Abrasive strips are then moved back and forth between the teeth to shape the actual sides of the teeth. Finally, the teeth are smoothed and polished.

Tooth contouring is quick, simple, painless, and inexpensive. This technique is most useful in cases of slight to moderate overlapping of the front teeth, slight rotation of the front teeth, uneven wear, or in cases where some teeth do not have their biting and incising edges in alignment. However, if teeth were uneven because of grinding, they will likely become uneven again if grinding is continued.

BRIDGES

If one or more teeth are missing, a difference in chewing and speaking may be noticed. Bridges help maintain the shape of the face, as well as alleviate the stress in the bite by replacing missing teeth. Sometimes called a fixed partial denture, a bridge replaces missing teeth with artificial teeth, looks natural, and literally bridges the gap where one or more teeth may have been.

The restoration can be made from gold, alloys, porcelain, or a combination of these materials and is bonded onto surrounding teeth for support. Unlike a removable bridge, which can be taken out and cleaned, a fixed bridge can only be removed by a dentist. An implant bridge attaches artificial teeth directly to the jaw or under the gum tissue. Depending on which type of bridge is recommended, its success depends on its foundation.

DENTURES

If natural teeth have been lost from periodontal disease, tooth decay, or injury, complete dentures can replace the missing teeth and the smile. Without support from the dentures, facial muscles sag, making a person look older. A conventional full denture is made and placed in the patient's mouth after the remaining teeth are removed and tissues have healed. This may take several months. A different type, known as an immediate complete denture, is inserted as soon as the remaining teeth are removed. With immediate dentures, teeth are not foregone during the healing period.

Dentures will seem awkward at first. When learning to eat, choose soft non-sticky food that is cut into small pieces, and chew slowly using both sides of the mouth.

In time, dentures need to be replaced or re-adjusted because of changes that occur in the tissues of the mouth. Brush the gums, tongue, and palate every morning with a soft-bristled brush before inserting the dentures. This will stimulate circulation in the tissues and help remove plaque. Keep dentures clean and free from food that can cause stains, bad breath, and gum irritation. Once a day, brush all surfaces of the dentures with a denture care product. Remove dentures from the mouth and place them in water or a denture cleansing liquid while sleeping. It is also helpful to rinse the mouth with a warm salt water solution in the morning, after meals, and at bedtime.

DENTAL IMPLANTS

Dental implants are anchors that permanently hold replacement teeth. Implants deliver artificial teeth that can be used to replace missing or decaying teeth, and for additional support combined with bridges, dentures, and crowns. They are an ideal alternative to a bridge if only one or a few teeth need to be replaced. Bridges attach artificial teeth to existing teeth, but implants attach directly to the jawbone or under the tissues of the gums. Implants are the most permanent way to replace missing teeth. Their main advantage is that they look and feel natural and fit very securely, which allows for better chewing ability and eliminates the embarrassment of dentures. The procedure is usually done in stages; surgery to position an anchor in the jaw to allow the bone to grow around may be followed by a second procedure to place a post-like fixture used to connect the anchor to the artificial teeth. Healthy gums and adequate bone are necessary to support the implant, and good oral hygiene is considered critical.

If there is not enough bone, a separate surgical procedure to add bone may be needed. Because bone heals slowly, treatment with implants can often take longer (four months to one year or more) to heal than bridges or dentures.

COSMETIC FILLINGS

To treat a cavity, the decayed portion of the tooth is removed and then the area on the tooth where the decayed material once lived is filled. Fillings are also used to repair cracked or broken teeth and teeth that have been worn down from misuse such as from nail-biting or tooth grinding.

Once the decay has been removed, the space is prepared for the filling by cleaning the cavity of bacteria and debris. If the decay is near the root, a liner made of glass ionomer, composite resin, or other material may be needed to protect the nerve. After the filling is in, it will be polished. Then the tooth-colored material is applied in layers and a special light that "cures" or hardens each layer is applied. When the multi-layering process is completed, the composite material is shaped to the desired result, excess material is trimmed and the final restoration is polished.

Today, several dental filling materials are available. Teeth can be filled with gold, porcelain, silver amalgam (which consists of mercury mixed with silver, tin, zinc, and copper), or tooth-colored plastic and glass materials called composite resin fillings. The location and extent of the decay, cost of filling material, will help determine the type of filling to best address individual needs.

COMPOSITE FILLINGS

With tooth-colored composite fillings, the shade and color of the composites can be closely matched to the color of existing teeth. These are particularly well-suited for use in front teeth or visible parts of teeth. Composite fillings actually chemically bond to tooth structure, providing further support to the tooth. In addition to use as a filling material for decay, composite fillings can also be used to repair chipped, broken, or worn teeth. Sometimes less tooth structure needs to be removed compared with amalgams when removing decay and preparing for the filling.

Composite fillings wear out sooner than amalgams (lasting at least five years compared to at least ten to fifteen years for amalgams). In addition, they may not last as long as amalgams under the pressure of chewing and particularly if used as the filling material for large cavities. Because of the process to apply the composite material, these fillings can take up to twenty minutes longer than amalgams to place. If composites are used for inlays or onlays, more than one office visit may be required. Depending on location, composite materials can chip off the tooth. Composite fillings can cost up to twice the cost of amalgams.

INLAYS AND ONLAYS

There are two types of indirect fillings: inlays and onlays. Inlays are similar to fillings but the entire work lies within the cusps (bumps) on the chewing surface of the tooth. Onlays are more extensive than inlays, covering one or more cusps. Onlays are sometimes called partial crowns. Inlays and onlays are more durable and last up to thirty years, much longer than traditional fillings. They can be made of tooth-colored composite resin, porcelain, or gold. Inlays and onlays weaken the tooth structure, but do so to a much lower extent than traditional fillings.

Another type of inlay and onlay, direct inlays and onlays, follow the same processes and procedures as the indirect, the difference is that direct inlays and onlays are made in the dental office and can be placed in one visit. The type of inlay or onlay used depends on how much sound tooth structure remains and consideration of any cosmetic concerns.

To maintain fillings, visit the dentist regularly for cleanings, brush with a fluoride-containing toothpaste, and floss at least once daily. If a filling might be cracked or is "leaking" (the sides of the filling do not fit tightly against the tooth, which allows debris and saliva to seep between the filling and the tooth), a dentist can take X-rays to assess the situation. If the tooth is extremely sensitive, if a sharp edge is felt, if you notice a crack in the filling is apparent, or if a piece of the filling is missing, call a dentist for an appointment.

SAFEGUARDING THE SMILE

Tooth Decay

Tooth decay is not just a children's disease; as long as teeth are in the mouth, they can decay. Tooth decay is caused by bacteria that cling to teeth and form a sticky, colorless film called dental plaque. The bacteria in plaque live on sugars and produce decay causing acids that dissolve minerals on tooth surfaces. Tooth decay can also develop on the exposed roots of the teeth if gum disease or receding gums (where gums pull away from the teeth, exposing the roots) is present.

Fluoride is important for adult teeth. Using fluoride toothpastes and mouth rinses can add protection. Daily fluoride rinses can be bought at most drug stores without a prescription. If cavities persist, a dentist or dental hygienist may give a fluoride treatment during the office visit. The dentist may prescribe a fluoride gel or mouth rinse to use at home.

Keeping Fillings in Good Shape

Constant pressure from chewing, grinding, or clenching can cause dental fillings to wear away, chip, or crack. If the seal between the tooth enamel and the filling breaks down, food particles and decay-causing bacteria can work their way under the filling. The risk of developing additional decay in that tooth is increased. Decay that is left untreated can progress to infect the dental pulp and may cause an abscessed tooth. If the filling is large or the recurrent decay is extensive, there may not be enough tooth structure remaining to support a replacement filling. In these cases, a dentist may need to replace the filling with a crown.

Gum Disease

A common cause of tooth loss after age thirty-five is gum (periodontal) disease. These are infections of the gum and bone that hold the teeth in place. Gum diseases are also caused by dental plaque. The bacteria in plaque causes the gums to become inflamed and bleed easily. If left untreated, the disease gets worse as pockets of infection form between the teeth and gums. This causes receding gums and loss of supporting bone. Enough bone may be lost to cause teeth to become loose and fall out. Gum disease can be prevented by removing plaque, and by thoroughly brushing and flossing every day. Carefully check for early signs of disease such as red, swollen, or bleeding gums.

Dry Mouth

Dry mouth or (xerostomia) can may make it hard to eat, swallow, taste, and speak. The condition happens when salivary glands fail to work properly as a result of various diseases or medical treatments, such as chemotherapy or radiation therapy to the head and neck area. Dry mouth is also a side effect of more than four hundred commonly used medicines, including drugs for high blood pressure, antidepressants, and antihistamines. Dry mouth can affect oral health by adding to tooth decay and infection. To relieve the dryness, drink extra water and avoid sugary snacks, beverages with caffeine, tobacco, and alcohol—all of which increase dryness in the mouth.

HEALTHY GUM TIPS FROM DR. LOWENBERG

- Brush teeth twice a day with fluoride toothpaste to remove decay-causing plaque

- Use a soft-bristled brush that fits the mouth and allows all areas to be easily reached

- Replace toothbrush every three to four months, or sooner if the bristles become frayed

- Clean between teeth daily with floss or an interdental cleaner. Decay causing bacteria still lingers between teeth where toothbrush bristles cannot reach. Flossing removes plaque and food particles from between the teeth and under the gum line

- Limit between-meal snacks, especially sweets and junk food

- Have professional cleanings and oral exams every three to four months.

BREATH APPEAL

Maintaining good oral health is essential to reduce bad breath. Regular professional cleanings help. Brush twice a day with fluoride toothpaste to remove food debris and plaque, and brush the tongue, too. Once a day, use floss or an interdental cleaner to clean between teeth. Mouthwashes do not have a long-lasting effect on bad breath. Products that contain both chlorine dioxide and zinc target the causes of bad breath. A fluoride mouth rinse, used along with brushing and flossing, can help prevent tooth decay.

Teeth are meant to last a lifetime. By taking good care of the teeth and gums, they can be protected for years to come. By taking care of the teeth and visiting the dentist regularly, healthy teeth and an attractive smile will always be there.

CHAPTER 12

Healthy Male
Check Up

The main reason why men do not see the doctor as often as women is because they subscribe to the theory; "If it ain't broke, don't fix it."

From the time we are little boys, guys are taught to be tough and not to cry or show emotion. That social training leads to middle-aged men ignoring chest pains that can warn of heart disease. Our culture prizes stoicism and courage among men, and it teaches men to be somewhat unresponsive to their own physical pain. Men tend to put their health aside because they are feeling well and are too busy to see the doctor. Or they may feel uncomfortable talking about their health problems. Or they just might not want to know if something is wrong. As a result, serious health problems may not emerge until they have reached a more advanced stage. While they may never consciously avoid going to the doctor, it is not a priority.

The Men's Health Network (MHN) reports that men die at higher rates than women from the top ten causes of death: heart disease, cancer, stroke, chronic obstructive pulmonary disease, accidents, pneumonia and influenza, diabetes, suicide, kidney disease, and chronic liver disease and cirrhosis. Men also die younger than women. In 1920, women outlived men only by one year. Today, CDC figures show the life expectancy gap has widened. On average, women survive men by six years. By the age of seventy-five, men die of cancer at approximately twice the rate of women.

BREAKING BAD HABITS

When a man is feeling well, he may not perceive any reason to see a doctor. They often do not visit a doctor on their own unless they have severe symptoms. It is less of a struggle to get women to see a doctor because women more often assume the role of caretaker and nurturer. Some men avoid going to the doctor because of fear—fear of finding out something is seriously wrong, and fear of having to take medications for a lifetime. Knowledge is one way to overcome that fear.

Men tend to have a "bulletproof" attitude toward their health. Women are far more likely than men to visit a doctor in general, although the gap narrows with increasing age. Traditionally, women research and select medical care for the family unit. However, that is changing rapidly. While men need to pay attention to their health, they also need to know where to go for help. Some in the healthcare field feel that the healthcare community in the United States does not do enough to reach out to men. Numerous programs alert women to the dangers of women's and children's health problems and actively encourage them to self-examine for female specific diseases and to have regular checkups. Yet, no effective program exists which is devoted to awareness and prevention of the leading killers of men. For male health care to improve, we have to get the word out to the male population and get them talking about their unique health needs. Many men do not know where to turn when they need help with gender-related concerns, such as finding a lump on a testicle or having trouble achieving an erection.

Another way to promote a long and healthy life is to partner up. Studies suggest that being married is healthful for men, as wives may prompt their husbands to take better care of themselves and to visit the doctor more regularly.

Start by going down the following checklist:

• **Compile a family history**—Knowing the health issues in one's family's past can help the patient and doctor better evaluate health habits and choose future medical treatments

• **Schedule screening tests**—Regular screening tests allow a doctor to learn what is typical, so it is easier to detect changes later in life. And these tests can help catch potential health problems early, when the odds for successful treatment are greatest

• **Get immunized**—Make sure all the immunizations are current. Find out when the last vaccination was against tetanus, diphtheria, measles, mumps, rubella, hepatitis A, hepatitis B, pneumonia, and influenza

TESTS TO HAVE AT EVERY AGE

Top Ten Male Health Risks

1. Heart Disease
2. Cancer
3. Unintentional Injuries

4. Stroke

5. Chronic obstructive pulmonary disease (COPD)

6. Diabetes

7. Influenza and Pneumonia

8. Suicide

9. Kidney Disease

10. Chronic liver disease and cirrhosis

Source: Centers for Disease Control and Prevention

All but one of these causes of death—stroke—claim proportionately more men's lives than women's lives at all ages. As a result, the average American man lives 5.4 years fewer than does the average woman. In 2002, male life expectancy was 74.5 years. Female life expectancy was 79.9 years.

It is unclear why men, statistically speaking, are the weaker sex. Heredity and male sex hormones may play a role, affecting such characteristics as body fat distribution. Specifically, men are more likely to accumulate fat around the abdomen (apple-shape obesity), which is associated with an increased risk of heart disease, diabetes, cancer, and stroke. Women, on the other hand, are more likely to put on extra weight around the hips. This pear-shape obesity, while unhealthy, is not linked as closely to potentially fatal conditions.

Socially sanctioned "male" behavior may also predispose men to premature death. Men are more likely to smoke, drink, use illicit drugs, and engage in casual sex—all of which can increase their risk of serious diseases. They are also conditioned from an early age to take risks and behave aggressively, which may partially explain why they have a higher risk of death from accidents, suicide, and homicide.

By recognizing the leading threats to life, one can take steps to reduce these risks.

Heart Disease

Heart disease presents a similar picture. It is the leading killer of men, and they are dying prematurely from heart disease at a much faster rate than women. The National Institute of Health has found that over three-quarters of all heart disease is related to diet and stress. Studies have attributed the higher death rate in men from heart disease to a lack of concern among men for their diets and the stress levels in their lives.

According to the MHN, almost twice as many males die of conditions that affect the cardiovascular system.

- According to the CDC, one in four men has some form of heart disease. It is the leading cause of death

- Average annual rates of the first heart disease complication rises from seven per 1,000 men at ages 35–44 to 68 per 1,000 at ages 85–94. For women, similar rates occur but they happen about 10 years later in life. The average age at which a person has a first heart attack is 65.8 for men and 70.4 for women

But heart disease does not just strike older men. Men have a shorter time to prevent the development of the condition so their overall risk is greater.

In addition to heart disease, stress also contributes to other disorders. For example, over 80 percent of those who suffer from peptic ulcers are men. The lack of concern for diet and stress has also affected men's sexual health. Sexually transmitted diseases, especially the continuing AIDS pandemic, are taking a frightening toll on young men.

Risk Factors for Heart Disease

- Increasing age
- Male sex
- Family history
- Ethnicity—African-Americans, Mexican Americans, Native Americans, Native Hawaiians, and some Asian Americans are at higher risk

- Smoking
- High cholesterol
- High blood pressure
- Physical inactivity
- Obesity
- Diabetes

Prostate Cancer

One in five men can expect to develop prostate cancer some time in his life. Thirty thousand American men will die from prostate cancer this year, and the numbers are continually increasing. It is the most common cancer found in men, the second leading type of cancer death in men, after lung cancer. Each year, approximately one hundred thousand new cases are reported. Although men who are diagnosed early on respond well to treatment, prostate cancer can be a painful killer if allowed to persist. While the early signs of prostate cancer are observable—for example, restricted flow of urine, pain in the prostate region or perineum, and later, sexual dysfunction—little education exists to teach men how to self-observe for this disease.

Men are not urged to undergo the simple digital examination that detects prostate disease. Studies have shown that the prostate digital exam is the test most frequently avoided or over-looked in a general health examination.

Every man over the age of forty should have a prostate examination at least every three years. Men over fifty should be examined every year. Unfortunately, only about 15 percent of men in this age group actually get examined annually.

Prostate cancer is not the only cancer that often goes undetected in men. Recent studies have shown that colon and rectal cancer are also prevalent among men and are often not detected early on. Also, men are not likely to perform self-examinations or seek tests for melanoma and other deadly forms of skin cancer. Because of a lack of awareness, poor health education, and the prevailing cultural stereotypes that discourage men from taking an active interest in their health, millions of men are dying unnecessarily early from cancers that could have been treated.

There is not enough known about what causes prostate cancer and how to prevent it. Yet the disease is treatable if found in early stages. This can be a challenge, since prostate cancer can show no symptoms until it has spread to other parts of the body.

The American Cancer Society (ACS) recommends an annual digital rectal exam and a prostate-specific antigen (PSA) test for healthy men fifty years or older. Men who have a family history of prostate cancer or who are African-American may want to ask their doctor about earlier testing.

Lung Cancer

Lung cancer is the leading cancer killer of both men and women, claiming more lives than prostate, colon, and breast cancer combined. In men, there are expected to be about 93,000 new cases of lung cancer and some 90,000 lung cancer deaths this year.

The good news is that rate of new lung cancer cases has been dropping since the 1980s, and deaths from the cancer have fallen since the 1990s as people are becoming increasingly aware of the harmful effects of tobacco.

Stroke

Stroke is the third leading killer in the country, after heart disease and all forms of cancer. The incidence rate of stroke is 1.25 times greater in men than in women, although there is really no difference between the sexes as people get older, according to the American Stroke Association.

Risk Factors

- Hypertension
- Increasing age
- African-Americans are at greater risk than whites.
- Gender, stroke is more common in men than in women until age 75
- Personal history of stroke or a transient ischemic attack (TIA, or ministroke)

- Diabetes
- High cholesterol
- Heart disease
- Smoking, including secondhand smoke
- Physical inactivity
- Obesity
- Alcohol and substance abuse

Depression

According to the National Institute of Mental Health, more than six million men experience depression each year. Men are four times more likely to commit suicide compared to women. Part of the blame can be attributed to underdiagnosed depression in men. Men are less likely to recognize the symptoms of depression, to openly show depression, or to have someone else recognize their emotional distress early enough to treat it.

Instead of sadness, depression may play out in the following ways in men:

- Anger
- Aggression
- Work "burnout"
- Risk-taking behavior
- Midlife crisis
- Alcohol and substance abuse

STAYING HEALTHY: OTHER CONCERNS MEN FACE

HEALTH CONCERN	INDICATIONS	PREVENTION	TREATMENT
STD	Transferred from one person to another through sexual contact, bodily fluids, and blood	Use condoms; if infected do not donate blood, organs, bone marrow, or semen	Most sexually transmitted diseases are treatable. However, even the once easily cured gonorrhea has become resistant to many of the older traditional antibiotics. Viral strains such as herpes, AIDS, and genital warts, have no cure
HEPATITIS C	Spread through contact with infected blood; damages liver	Do not share toothbrushes, razors, or other personal care items; cover your cuts and open sores; use disinfectants and bandages when dressing cuts and wounds; practice safe sex by using latex condoms; do not donate blood, organs, bone marrow, or semen; let anyone who could come into contact with your blood know, including sexual partners, doctors, or dentists	Interferon reduces liver inflammation, Ribavirin helps prevent the virus from multiplying. Stop drinking alcohol and using recreational injection drugs; eat a healthy diet and exercise; get vaccinated against hepatitis A and hepatitis B; check with your doctor about other prescription drugs you may be using; get a liver biopsy
ERECTILE DYSFUNCTION	Damage to nerves, arteries, smooth muscles, and fibrous tissues, often resulting from diseases; surgery; injury to the penis, spinal cord, prostate, bladder, and pelvis; common medicines such as blood pressure drugs, antihistamines, antidepressants, tranquilizers, appetite suppressants, and cimetidine; psychological factors; smoking; hormonal abnormalities (low testosterone)		sildenafil citrate (Viagra), vardenafil hydrochloride, Levitra, Cialis

PROSTATE CANCER	Unknown; the growth of cancer cells in the prostate, like that of normal prostate cells, is stimulated by male hormones, especially testosterone	Prostate cancer screening, including a digital rectal examination (DRE) and test to measure prostate-specific antigen (PSA) in the blood, should be taken yearly after the age of 50; men with two or more first-degree relatives affected by the disease or those of African-American descent should consider starting prostate cancer screenings at an earlier age	Prostatectomy (removal of the prostate);hormonal/ drug therapy; radiation therapy; Orchiectomy (surgical removal of the testes which results in impotence); chemotherapy; Dutasteride
SCROTAL MASSES	Can signal something as serious as testicular cancer or may indicate a less serious or harmless condition (such as fluid accumulation, an infection, an extended hernia, or varicose veins)		The hernia sac and swelling can be removed with a surgical procedure; testicular cancer requires surgery
EPIDIDYMITIS	Infection and swelling of the epididymis, the male organ that collects and delivers sperm; a sperm cyst (spermatocele)		Antibiotics
INGUINAL HERNIA	Can extend into your scrotum and cause a swelling above the testicle		Surgical repair
VARICOCELE	A collection of prominent (varicose) veins in the spermatic cord above your testicle; may cause infertility; swelling may increase after heavy lifting or exercise and decrease on lying down		Surgical treatment usually is not necessary unless an infertility problem is present

TESTS TO HAVE AT EVERY AGE

SCREENING TESTS: WHAT YOU NEED AND WHEN

If you ask a woman why breast exams are necessary, she will most likely know the answer. However, if you ask a man why testicular exams are needed, he will most likely dismiss the idea as not necessary, or keep postponing the exam.

To maintain health and detect problems early on, men need to undergo a routine physical exam every year after the age of eighteen. This exam should include relevant screening tests. A screening test such as a colorectal cancer test is recommended to detect cancers and other diseases early on, while they are easier to treat. The frequency and type of test varies from man to man, depending on medical history, family history, and lifestyle.

What tests do you need?

TYPE OF TEST	WHAT IT SCREENS FOR	AGE TO START REGULAR TESTING	FREQUENCY
Blood Pressure	High blood pressure, hypertension, kidney disease, strokes	21	Annually, more often if over 140/90
Cholesterol	Cholesterol count of the blood	35 (if you smoke, have diabetes, or if heart disease runs in your family, start at 20)	Every 5 years
Colorectal Exam Fecal Occult Blood Test Colonoscopy DRE Double-Contrast Barium Enema	Colorectal cancer	40	Depends on type of test: Fecal Occult Blood Test: annually Colonoscopy: every 5 years DRE: every 5 years Double-Contrast Barium Enema: every 5 to 10 years

Dental Exam	Cavities, gum disease, other oral problems	18	Every 6 months or as directed
Diabetes	Elevated blood sugar	Any age	Once a year
Electrocardiogram	Heart attacks and abnormal heart rhythms	18	As directed
Eye Exam	Cataracts, glaucoma, visual acuity	As needed	Baseline exam every two to four years
PSA Blood Test/ Digital Rectal Exam	Prostate cancer	50	Annually (earlier if you have a family history of prostate cancer or are African American
Sexually Transmitted Diseases	HIV, chlamydia, gonorrhea, herpes, etc.	If sexually active	As needed
Testicular Self-Exam	Painless lumps that indicate testicular cancer; hold each testicle between the thumb and fingers of both hands and gently roll to check for any abnormal lumps	15	Monthly, after a shower or bath
Tuberculosis Skin Test	Tuberculosis bacteria	18	As directed
Breast Cancer	Check breast for lumps		Total body skin exam by dermatologist: 3 years Chest X-ray: 5 years

TESTOSTERONE

In response to the growing desire to stay young and live longer, researchers are exploring hormonal substances that will increase the lifespan. Although the solution to eternal youth and longevity is probably not testosterone, the full range of its potential is underappreciated. Along with twenty years of clinical experience, current research findings suggest that testosterone replacement may improve the quality of life in older men. Studies have confirmed that as men age, even if they are in good health, their testosterone levels decrease. It is currently believed that the decrease of testosterone is caused by the failure of the gonadotropin-releasing hormone pulse generator along with a malfunction in the pituitary gland.

The Role of Testosterone

Sexual Function

Numerous studies have demonstrated a strong correlation between testosterone and sexual behavior. Testosterone levels, however, relate more strongly to the libido than to erections. In order for sildenafil (Viagra) to be effective, studies have shown that men must have an adequate testosterone level in order to sustain an erection, possibly because of its effects on nitric oxide synthetase.

Memory Effects

There is a strong relationship between testosterone and performance on a number of different memory tests.

Strength

Several studies have correlated testosterone with physical strength and muscle function. Two of these studies demonstrated that administering testosterone improved upper grip strength. A decrease in testosterone will cause a decline in muscle mass.

Bone Density

The level of testosterone also affects the resilience of bones. Studies have shown that testosterone affects lumbar spine density. Other studies have proven that death from hip fractures is higher in men with a low level of testosterone.

Blood Composition

Studies have shown that the ratio of red blood cells to whole blood increases with testosterone supplements. Testosterone has been linked to this increase since the hemoglobin in women does not decline as they age. For men undergoing testosterone replacement, blood must be checked every four to six months to make sure that the ratio of red blood cells to whole blood does not become too high.

Prostate Cancer

No clinical evidence has demonstrated that the risk of prostate cancer increases with testosterone replacement.

Cardiovascular Risk

The lower the level of testosterone in an individual, the more likely he is to have coronary artery disease. This connection has been known since the 1940s when testosterone was used to treat angina. Data also suggests that testosterone relaxes the coronary arteries by liberating nitric oxide, an effect very similar to that of estrogen.

THE NATURAL DECLINE OF TESTOSTERONE

Starting around age forty, a man's body produces about one percent less testosterone each year. Testosterone is the main male hormone that maintains muscle mass and strength, fat distribution, bone mass, sperm production, sex drive, and potency.

Many call this progressive decline of hormones "male menopause" or "andropause" and equate it to women's menopause. In women, ovulation ceases and female hormone production plummets over a relatively short time frame. In men, there's a gradual decline in the production of male hormones.

For most men, testosterone levels naturally decline but still remain within the normal range throughout their lifetime, causing no significant problems. About two in 10 men age 60 and older have testosterone levels below the normal range (testosterone deficiency).

Testosterone deficiency can have several effects on the body:

- Decreased energy
- Reduced muscle mass and strength
- Decreased cognitive function
- Less sexual interest or potency
- Depressed mood

If you experience these signs or symptoms, you may or may not have testosterone deficiency. Other medical conditions—such as liver disease, hypothyroidism and depression—can cause these effects as can certain medications, including beta blockers, pain killers and certain drugs for depression or anxiety. In addition, some healthy men encounter these changes as a part of the natural aging process, possibly because of declining hormones other than testosterone.

What Is Male Menopause?

Male menopause, also called viropause or andropause, begins with hormonal, physiological, and chemical changes that occur in all men between the ages of forty and fifty-five. However, it can occur as early as thirty-five and as late as sixty-five. These changes affect all aspects of a man's life. Male menopause is a physical condition with psychological, interpersonal, social, and emotional dimensions.

Although the causes of male menopause have not been fully researched, there are several factors known to contribute to this condition. They include hormone deficiencies, excessive alcohol consumption, smoking, hypertension, prescription and non-prescription medications, poor diet, lack of exercise, poor circulation, and psychological problems. It is also known that male menopause is a syndrome associated with a lack of or absence of testosterone. A general decline in male potency at mid-life can be expected in most men. Even in healthy men, the amount of testosterone secreted into the bloodstream at age fifty-five is significantly lower than it was ten years earlier. By age eighty, most male hormone levels have decreased to pre-puberty levels. There are two general forms of male menopause found in adult men who had normal hormone levels through puberty and young adulthood and who experienced normal sexual development.

SCREENING AND TESTING FOR TESTOSTERONE DEFICIENCY
You may suffer from testosterone deficiency if you answer yes to any of the following questions.
Do you have a decrease in libido or sex drive?
Do you have a lack of energy?
Do you have a decrease in strength or endurance?
Have you noticed any significant weight loss?
Do you feel that you have lost your enjoyment in life?
Are you sad or grumpy?
Are your erections less strong?
Has your ability to participate in sports declined?
Do you fall asleep right after dinner?
Has your performance at work deteriorated recently?

Testosterone replacement given at the time of "andropause" (the male equivalent to menopause) has shown increases in libido, memory, strength, and the ratio of red blood cells to whole blood. In addition to the research data, clinical experience has demonstrated that testosterone in replacement dosage may improve quality of life and function in middle-aged and older men. Recent studies have also demonstrated a link between testosterone production and Alzheimer's.

Testosterone Therapy

The possibilities are enticing: Increase muscle mass, sharpen memory and mental focus, boost libido, and improve energy level. If an older man, this may sound like the ultimate anti-aging formula. But the benefits touted from testosterone therapy are not quite so clear cut.

Testosterone therapy has been used successfully for years to treat men with abnormally low testosterone levels—a medical condition called male hypogonadism. More recently, healthy, aging men have taken the hormone to boost waning testosterone levels. But not enough is known about the effects of testosterone therapy for this purpose. No long-term studies have weighed the potential benefits against the possible risks, including infertility and prostate problems.

Testosterone therapy appears to be growing in popularity. At the core of the controversy is whether gradually declining testosterone levels are a natural phenomenon or a health condition, and whether it should be treated.

Benefits & Risks of Testosterone Therapy

In hypogonadal men, testosterone therapy can restore sexual function and muscle strength and prevent bone loss. Some men taking testosterone therapy report an increase in energy and sex drive.

Some anti-aging enthusiasts claim that increasing the level of testosterone in older and healthy men provides these same benefits. High doses of testosterone may result in sleeping problems, infertility, and excess blood production, which could increase the risk of stroke. Increasing testosterone levels may also pose problems for the prostate, a small male gland that produces most of the fluids in semen.

Testosterone naturally stimulates the growth of the prostate. Long-term testosterone treatment could cause benign prostatic hyperplasia (BPH)—enlargement of the prostate gland. This is a concern that testosterone therapy might fuel the growth of prostate cancer that is already present. Prostate cancer is increasingly common in older men, and many men have prostate cancer that is not diagnosed. Testosterone therapy is clearly beneficial for men whose testicles fail to produce sufficient levels of testosterone (hypogonadism). For this group of men, it can restore sexual function and muscle strength and prevent bone loss.

In November 2003, the Institute of Medicine (IOM) reviewed the current evidence surrounding testosterone therapy and reported that this treatment is only appropriate for men who produce little or no testosterone. The IOM concluded that the long-term effects of supplemental testosterone on otherwise healthy men are not known. Until more studies have been done, the IOM recommends that testosterone therapy not be used to prevent or relieve the physical or psychological effects of aging.

JUMPSTARTING YOUR WORKOUT PLAN

"I teach the Super Slow Technique because it improves strength at any age. The combination of slow movement, steady breathing, and isolating muscle groups strengthens joints and minimizes the pressure placed on them. It is a wonderful regimen to improve bone density and combat arthritis as you mature."—David Finley, personal trainer

The Energy Decade: The 20s

Think of the twenties as a decade of pregame practice. Invest a couple of hours of effort every week, and it will help by slowing down decline later on.

Perform this workout two days a week.

Do two or three sets of six to eight repetitions, starting with a weight that is about 30 percent to 50 percent of the one-rep max for the throws and squats, and 70 percent to 85 percent for the other exercises. Perform the throws and jump squats as fast as possible; for the others, take two seconds up, four seconds down.

- Jump squat
- Bench-press throw (on Smith machine)
- Straight-bar biceps curl
- Stiff-legged deadlift

- Shoulder press
- Lat pulldown
- Hanging knee raise (work up to 20 reps)

Prevention and Planning: The 30s

The physiological capacity—the overall performance of most of the body's systems—decreases by around 1 percent per year from age thirty onward. To counter this physiological decline, switch the strategy to preventive fitness. Continue lifting heavy weights to preserve the muscle built in the twenties; stretching takes priority, because flexibility will decrease. Regular interval training is on the list to combat the loss of stamina that will start in the middle of this decade. It is never too late to make a fresh start.

Perform this workout two or three days a week.

Do two or three sets of eight to ten repetitions, starting with 75 percent of the one-rep maximum. If more than twelve reps are possible, then lift more weight. If form worsens before ten reps, use a lighter weight. The tempo for all of these is two seconds up, four seconds down.

- **Dumbbell lunge**—You will put less strain on your knees if you take large steps and make sure your front knee is lined up directly over (not past) your toes
- **Cable fly**—Bend forward slightly from the hips and keep the shoulders pressed down and back
- **Seated leg curl**—Do not allow the back to lift off the pad
- **Bent-over row**—Tighten the abs, bend at the hips, and keep the back flat
- **Reverse curl**—Do not bring the forearm beyond perpendicular to the floor

Never Back Down: The 40s

During the forties, it becomes apparent that the body's warranty has indeed expired. The forties are also when career is established, so late-night duty is for junior staff. For the first time since college, discretionary time is an option. You have earned three hours of workout time during the week and a longer session on the weekends. No excuses. The body needs the work right now; delay is not an option.

Perform this workout two days a week.

Do two or three sets of ten to twelve reps, starting with 70 percent of the one-rep max. If more than twelve reps are possible, lift more weight. If form is lost before twelve reps, use a lighter weight. Take two seconds going up, six seconds down.

• Barbell squat	• Incline biceps curl
• Dumbbell bench press	• Standing calf raise
• Dumbbell shoulder press (or Arnold press)	• Russian twist (start with 15 reps to each side; build up to 25)
• Seated row	

Defending Turf: 50 and Beyond

By now a man has it figured out. He is a master at the office, a veteran in the weight room, the head of the family, but he is fighting Mother Nature and it is an uphill battle.

Performing at least two exercise sessions per week boosts a man's self-esteem by helping him feel better about his body's ability to perform routine tasks. Feeling good also motivates you to make more gains. A fitness program should help avoid pain and do what is important.

Perform this workout two days a week.

Do two or three sets of ten to fifteen repetitions, starting with 65 percent of your one-rep max. If more than fifteen reps are possible, lift more weight. If form is lost before ten reps, use a lighter weight. Keep the speed at six seconds up, six seconds down.

- One-legged half squat (begin without weight)
- One-legged deadlift (with or without weight)
- One-arm row (on low cable pulley)
- Lateral raise and front raise
- Standing alternating arm curl
- Lying dumbbell pullover
- Standing overhead medicine-ball throw (against a wall or with a partner)

CHAPTER 13

Living Longer
& Healthier

"Without exercise, any discussion on controlling weight comes to a screeching halt. Trying to lose weight permanently through food manipulation alone has been shown over and over to be a worthless, antiquated approach."

– David Finley

Healthy Eating

You have tried the low carb diet, and counting calories takes too much time. Trying to lose weight without increasing physical activity is simply a bust all by itself. You have to become fit and train to achieve fat loss. The most successful means of controlling weight and fat is a combination of sensible eating and fitness.

The National Center for Health Statistics has found that about 25 percent of Americans get almost no exercise at all, which increases chances of having a heart attack, diabetes, and cancer. One in four adults with an advanced degree do high levels of exercise, compared with only one in seven with less than a high school diploma. Men are also more likely to exercise than women. The poorer you are, the less exercise you do.

OZ GARCIA'S TOP FIVE POWER FOODS FOR MEN

Blueberries

Make blueberries part of the diet. Blueberries are recognized as being one of world's healthiest foods, ranking number one in antioxidant activity when compared to forty other fresh fruits and vegetables. Anthocyanin, the pigment that makes the blueberries blue, is thought to be responsible for the high content of antioxidants that offer major health benefits. The strong amount of antioxidants in blueberries helps neutralize "free radicals" that can lead to cancer and other age related diseases. Most impressive is the ability of blueberries to improve memory as well as undo some degenerative changes seen in aging neurons. Over the past year, scientists tested blueberries against an array of common disorders and discovered significant results. One study showed that blueberries were effectual in suppressing free radical and inflammatory damage in the brain. Another showed that blueberries may reduce the build up of so called "bad" cholesterol that contributes to cardiovascular disease and stroke. As well, a compound was found in blueberries that promotes urinary tract health and reduces the risk of infection. Blueberries have even been linked with improving eyesight and helping ease eye fatigue.

Salmon

Omega-3 fatty acids are in the oil naturally found in fish. Of all fish, salmon contains the highest amounts of omega-3. New studies about omega-3 fatty acids are so impressive that the federal government has stated that fish oil can help save lives. The omega-3 fats, EPA and DHA, play different but equally vital roles in human health. EPA helps make the platelets in blood less sticky which in turn could help prevent the build-up of plaque otherwise leading to a heart attack or stroke. DHA may help stabilize heart rhythm; potentially important for people recovering from heart attacks. As well, it helps regulate cell membrane functions involved in transmitting signals among brain cells. In Chicago's Western Electric Study (over 2,000 men) the risk of death from heart attack was half the usual rate among those who ate an average of about eight ounces of fish (two servings) a week. Other recent research suggests that just one serving a week of "fattier" fish, like salmon or mackerel, could cut the chance of cardiac arrest by 50 percent in folks with weakened hearts. Omega-3 have been reported to help relieve joint pain and morning stiffness caused by rheumatoid arthritis. The American College of Rheumatology recommends eating fish more often. Omega-3 are also recognized for supporting healthy brain function.

These fats may be helpful in mood and brain disturbances. Fish oil may also be helpful in lowering blood triglyceride levels in patients with high blood levels. Last but not least, Omega-3 suppress tumor growth in animals, which may prove beneficial to humans, as well.

Pomegranate

Used in folk medicine to treat inflammation, sore throats, and rheumatism for centuries, the pomegranate has recently been rediscovered and acclaimed for its health benefits, in particular, for its disease-fighting antioxidant potential. Preliminary studies suggest that pomegranate juice may contain almost three times the total antioxidant ability compared with the same quantity of green tea or red wine. It also provides a substantial amount of potassium, is high in fiber, and contains vitamin C and niacin. Scientists have shown that drinking a daily glass of the fruit's juice can reduce the risk of cardiovascular as it slows down cholesterol oxidation by almost half, and reduces the retention of LDL. Pomegranate has substances that have antioxidant, anti-viral, and anti-tumor activity and compounds that play a role in prostate and osteoarthritis health.

Walnuts and Pecans

Walnuts and Pecans are as nutritious to eat as they are delicious. These nuts are excellent sources of protein and contain energy producing nutrients. Walnuts and pecans are cholesterol-free and contain healthy, unsaturated fats which can help lower the risk of heart disease. They also provide polyphenols and resveratrol, the most effective plant extract for maintaining optimal health. Resveratrol may help to prevent the effects of cardiac fibrosis. Researchers also believe that the resveratrol found in walnuts and pecans could also protect against age-related macular degeneration. Walnuts and pecans also provide iron, calcium, vitamins A, B, and C, potassium, and phosphorous. These nuts also contain magnesium, which helps maintain bone structure and chromium, which helps to ensure proper insulin function. They contain zinc for growth and wound healing and manganese, which protects against free radicals. All nuts are a good source of vitamin E, an important antioxidant. Like all plant foods, they are high in fiber and phytochemicals—both of which help protect against cancer and other chronic diseases.

Recent studies have shown that a small serving of these nuts four times per a week has been observed to reduce the risk of cardio vascular disease and help to lower blood cholesterol, levels, reduce oxidation of low density lipoprotein (LDL) cholesterol and improve a number of other related to cardiovascular disease. Nuts have often had bad press, being called "a fatty food" to be avoided by those trying to reduce or control their weight. Two recent studies have shown eating a reasonable amount of nuts in the diet does not lead to weight gain.

Red Wine

In Greek and Roman mythology there were gods and goddesses of wine ,and Plato may have been wiser than he knew when he said, "Nothing more excellent or valuable than wine was ever granted by the gods to man." Those of us who have come to enjoy the variety and tastes that wine have to offer can now look to red wines for greater health benefits.

Recent studies indicate that moderate red wine consumption may help protect against certain cancers, heart disease, and lower inflammation, and can have a positive effect on cholesterol levels and blood pressure. Polyphenols are antioxidant compounds found in the skin and seeds of grapes. Resveratrol is a type of plyphenol produced as part of a plant's defense system against disease. It is produced in the plant in response to an invading fungus, stress, injury, infection, or ultraviolet irradiation. Red wine contains high levels of resveratrol.

OZ GARCIA'S TOP 5 SUPPLEMENTS FOR MEN

Gamma Tocopherol

It is only in the last decade that the public began to be educated about the critical fact that "vitamin E" is not a single compound. Instead, it is a general name for a whole family of compounds. Eight forms of vitamin E have been identified. These powerful forms of Vitamin E belong either to the tocopherol sub-family or to the tocotrienol sub-family. The scientific focus is slowly shifting away from "vitamin E" to specific tocopherols and tocotrienols.

It turns out that the heretofore neglected beta, gamma, and delta tocopherols and tocotrienols seem to have important health benefits, including anti-inflammatory, cardioprotective, and anticancer activity. Gamma tocopherol in particular also has the ability to protect against nitrogen-based free radicals, which alpha tocopherol cannot do. Nitrogen free radicals play an important role in diseases associated with chronic inflammation, including cancer, heart disease, and degenerative brain disorders such as Alzheimer's disease. Studies also show that men with the highest levels of gamma tocopherol had only one-fifth the risk of prostrate cancer compared with the men with the lowest levels.

Folic Acid

Folic acid has been known to exert a protective effect against cardiovascular diseases, some forms of cancer, and various neurological impairments. Folate is necessary for cell replication and growth, as well as the synthesis of DNA and RNA, the cell's genetic blueprints. Folate helps prevent alterations to DNA that can lead to cancer. It is unfortunately, estimated that 88 percent of all North Americans suffer from a folic acid deficiency. Folic acid deficiency has been implicated in a wide variety of disorders from Alzheimer's disease to atherosclerosis, heart attack, stroke, osteoporosis, cervical and colon cancer, depression, dementia, cleft lip and palate, hearing loss, and neural tube defects.

Acetyl L Carnitine

Acetyl-L-carnitine is a molecular compound found in the brain, kidneys, and liver. This substance is also artificially produced as a dietary supplement. Acetyl-L-carnitine is a natural remedy super antioxidant that has been shown in clinical studies to benefit cognitive ability, memory, and mood. Acetyl-L-carnitine assists in enabling dietary fats to be converted to energy and muscle. Acetyl-L-carnitine has also been suggested as a possible neuroprotective agent that may also be useful for strokes, Down's syndrome, and for the management of various neuropathies. Based on successful studies, some scientists claim that acetyl-L-carnitine may be a helpful supplement for people with a loss of muscular coordination caused by disease in the cerebellum. Acetyl-L-Carnitine may have certain anti-aging properties and there is promising research to support the beneficial effect acetyl-l-carnitine has on sperm movement.

DHEA

DHEA is a necessary building block for a variety of compounds manufactured in the human body. Levels of DHEA, a natural pro-hormone in the body, have been shown to peak between ages twenty and thirty and then decrease progressively with age. It is believed that as we age the progressive deficiency of this hormone may be associated with the symptoms of aging. DHEA increases lean muscle, protects the immune system, is a precursor to testosterone, and helps burn fat. In a recent study, participants who took DHEA had more energy, slept better, and handled stress better than the placebo-takers. DHEA increases the body's ability to transform food into energy, burn off excess fat, and prevent fat from accumulating in the first place. DHEA has been proven to have a significant impact on fat loss and lean muscle mass and has also been shown to block some acute effects of stress induced cortisol release during exercise.

Colostrum

It is likely that colostrum was the very first nourishment received after being born. Colostrum is an enriched balance of powerful antibodies, proteins, antioxidants, immunoglobulins, growth factors, minerals, enzymes, amino acids, and essential vitamins specially designed to ensure the survival of the newborn. Colostrum's nutritional factors are astounding and are only possible from nature. Colostrum supplementation fortifies the immune system. If a boost to a healthy immune system is desired or a compromised immune system is present, colostrum may be the answer. Colostrum can jump-start the need to fight infection or immune-related chronic diseases such as cancer.

AEROBICS & BELT SIZE

"Staying fit is the best medicine in the world—it is the key to a longer, more quality life. The true fountain of youth is good fitness training, a balanced diet, proper sleep, and managing your level."—Dave Finley

Aerobic exercise turns out to be critical in the management of the hunger mechanism, and the storage of fat in cells. It helps to keep you in the lower range of your setpoint, controlling insulin levels in blood, and helping your body accurately adjust caloric intake to output.

Exercise changes the way the body processes food, making it easier for it to be used for energy than to be stored as fat. When you are active, the fat in a meal tends to be burned for energy. When you are sedentary, the amount of fat that's burned goes way down and winds up being stored (in all the wrong places) instead of being used by the muscles.

Best Forms of Aerobic Activity

- Walking
- Running
- Spinning
- Cycling

- Hiking
- Aerobic classes
- Skiing

Exercise is aerobic if it makes the heart and lungs work harder to meet the muscles' need for oxygen. Aerobic exercise uses the lower part of the body, thighs, and buttocks because the larger the muscle is, the greater the volume of calories that are burned.

How much exercise is appropriate? Most experts suggest thirty to forty-five minutes of moderately intense activity (like vigorous walking) every day. When exercising aerobically, try to work up to a heart rate between 130 and 150 beats a minute, depending on age (if young, go for the higher heart rate; as you age, the goal is the lower number). This is your target heart rate (HRT). Reaching it, and keeping it there for thirty to forty-five minutes, will put you into your fat-burning mode.

Adding muscle through weight training is a second and necessary tool for weight control. Weight training is an example of anaerobic exercise, which does not need extra oxygen. This type of exercise uses up the food stored in the muscles quickly, often within three or four minutes. Some men are afraid to pursue weight training because they think it will make them gain additional pounds. Weight training develops lean body mass (muscle); the more lean mass present, the faster the metabolism. For men trying to drop weight and looking to maintain their lean muscle mass as they get older (this accounts for all of us), weight training is essential because:

• Muscle tissue is seventy times more metabolically active than fat

• Muscle uses far more calories than the same amount of fat tissue

• Muscle is the most energy-active tissue in the body

• Fat is burned more efficiently for every additional pound of muscle. For every pound of new muscle put on, fifty to one hundred more calories will be burned per day

Get Professional Help

It is difficult to make universal recommendations for starting a muscle-building, strengthening, or toning program. If possible, seek out professional advice and coaching. Get a trainer, do it right. A personal trainer does not have to be present at every workout. Find someone who will work two or three times to help determine the best workout for your goals and current fitness level. This will minimize injuries and maximize gains.

It becomes more difficult to lose weight as one ages for several reasons. About one half pound of muscle is naturally lost each year after the age of twenty-five (if you do not stay fit). That is about five or six pounds each decade, so that by age fifty-six you have lost 25 to 30 percent of your muscle mass and strength. And you know what will fill up all that space: fat!

Sleep and Stress Control

The amount of sleep has a direct correlation to weight gain. Numerous studies have linked a failure to receive adequate sleep, especially a part of the sleep called rapid eye movement (REM) sleep, with weight gain. In an apparently vicious cycle, sleep problems can contribute to weight gain and obesity—and weight gain and obesity can interfere with sleep.

If overly tired during the day, wake up at night, and told that you snore, consider the possibility that of have sleep apnea. Nearly 40 percent of the population has sleep apnea, a condition where one actually stops breathing several times during the night. It is often coupled with severe snoring. Sleep apnea contributes to weight gain, at least in part by disrupting REM sleep. It also causes fatigue and may spur heart disease and other serious illnesses. Treatments for sleep apnea include CPAP (a mask that blows air through the nose while sleeping), dental devices, surgery to hold airways open, and monitoring breathing in a professional sleep laboratory. By the time men reach the age of forty-five, they have nearly lost the ability to fall into deep sleep.

Silencing Snoring

Snoring can be caused by many factors. The key to overcoming it is to find the underlying cause. Snoring can be related to other sleeping disorders such as narcolepsy and sleep apnea. It can also be due to a physical condition such as enlarged adenoids, a deviated septum, or broken nose.

To alleviate snoring, try sleeping without a pillow, adopt a healthier diet, and cut out smoking, sleeping pills and alcohol. If snoring is caused by allergies, antihistamines or a nasal decongestant might help. On the more extreme end, corrective surgery of internal nasal airway obstruction may be advised.

MONITORING STRESS

Another essential goal is controlling stress. Here is another chicken-and-egg conundrum: stress influences the food eaten, and the food eaten influences stress. An increase in appetite might be experienced when you are stressed out. If so, you may be suffering from hyperglycemia, or high blood sugar. Your cortisol levels may be high. Essentially, the body is accessing and burning the fuel available in the food you are eating, rather than properly accessing stored fat. When that happens, you try to keep yourself energized by eating sugar and carbs.

On the other hand, stress may cause you to eat less often, albeit in larger meal portions. That might be a sign that stress is making your thyroid and adrenal glands sluggish, and slowing down your metabolic activity. You may also look to sugar and caffeine to keep yourself going.

Whatever your reaction, stress and stress-based eating cause disturbances in a hormone called cholecystokinin (CCK), the substance that signals the brain to make you feel full. When you are under stress, you tend to eat faster. Therefore, you do not give CCK enough time to send its signals to the brain. Your stoplight system is out of order, and you will eat more than you should.

Sitting back and taking supplements alone is not going to do it for you. Supplements should be used as part of a supervised weight management program.

If you have severe weight problems and have experienced no results from all the other components listed in this chapter, talk to your doctor about the possibility of using prescription drugs although this should not be your first line of defense.

If we ate like our ancestors did, we would be better protected from diseases including heart disease, adult-onset diabetes, and many types of cancer. We love to eat—which is important for our survival—but apparently we will eat just about anything, regardless of whether or not it is good for us.

Will power simply does not stand a chance when our ancestral instincts are telling us that we had better eat as much as we can before the famine sets in—and when this new convenience-food environment makes it so easy for us to do so.

What Is the Food/Hormone Connection?

Our ancestors did not have the kinds of food choices we have today. They did not have breads, pastas, grains, and sugar-laden desserts. If they craved sweets, it was because they needed the vitamin C that fruits and berries provided. Whatever they consumed worked efficiently with their bodies' own chemistry.

The problem with today's modern diet is that huge amounts of sugar and processed carbohydrates wreak havoc on our health. These food substances adversely affect chemicals, known as hormones, which are our bodies' biological messengers. They tell our organs, cells, and tissues what to do and when to do it. The hormonal (or endocrine) system is one of the body's great communication networks. Hormones are involved in just about every biological process: immune function, reproduction, growth, even controlling other hormones. Even minute doses of harmful substances may serve to disrupt the body's efficiency level.

Hormonal Control

There are three key things you can do to control your hormones:

1. Watch what you eat

2. Get enough exercise

3. Reduce stress

The result will be the potential to control everything from the restoring and managing of strength, muscle mass, stamina, and sexuality, to decreasing the risk of degenerative illnesses.

FOODS THAT DE-STRESS

Any kind of fruit is fine; the sugar in it gives the little burst of energy that the adrenaline-charged body is craving. But go for oranges in particular. Most men become manually or orally fixated when they are stressed out—that is why some men smoke, and others fail to notice they chomped through a whole can of Pringles two innings ago. Peeling an orange will keep the hands and mouth busy.

SIMPLIFYING SUPPLEMENTS

According to the USDA—which analyzed the diets of thousands of men— the average male is woefully low on certain important dietary vitamins and minerals even if he takes a multivitamin pill. Focus on getting more calcium, folate, and vitamin E—key nutrients for bone, heart, and immune-system health.

NUTRIENT	AMOUNT YOU NEED
Calcium	1,000 mg
Magnesium	410 mg
Phosphorus	700 mg
Folate	400 mcg
Niacin	16 mg
Riboflavin	1.3 mg
Thiamin	1.2 mg
Vitamin B6	1.3 mg
Vitamin B12	2.4 mcg
Vitamin C	90 mg
Vitamin E	15 mg

STRESS REDUCTION

YOGA

Yoga builds bodies that are strong and supple, soft and toned, rather than hard or tense. Practicing any yoga posture in a relaxing way with slow deep breathing and letting go may relax the nervous system. Learning to relax and reduce stress through meditation may even help to reduce the risk of heart attack and stroke.

Yoga has three components:

- Postures or stretches designed to lengthen, strengthen and relax the body
- Breathing exercises that help to relax and cleanse the body, which promote healthy skin, muscle tone, and a lengthened, strong body
- Philosophy that teaches the mind to relax and to eliminate chaos and distractions

The mission of yoga is to align the heart, body, mind, and spirit, which will ultimately bring a sense of inner tranquility. Getting enough rest and sleep is another important part of sticking to the plan. Exhaustion and stress will wear down the immune system, and take their toll on one's energy level.

Everything that affects the skin affects the body, and vice versa. The skin is connected to the brain, the nervous system, the hormones, and the immune system. In broader terms, the mind-skin link reflects health as well as disease.

FEEL GOOD FACTOR

Keep in mind that the whole body is interrelated. If any aspect, physical or mental is neglected, the system goes out of kilter to either a greater or lesser degree. Feeling good about yourself translates to a positive mind-body connection. In other words, relaxation is the remedy for stress and tension. The aim is relaxation of the entire system, both body and mind. When muscles are totally at ease, circulation is equalized and the body can function at an optimum level. In addition, massages, breathing exercises, and physical activity will help the body relax. Perhaps the oldest relaxation therapy is great sex.

THE BENEFITS OF MASSAGE

Massage calms the nerve receptors in the skin, decreases blood pressure and pulse rate, promotes removal of lactic acid in the muscles, and induces deeper breathing and a sense of well-being.

Deep Massage Exercise

Begin by gently stroking with moderate, firm, light heavy pressure, taking care not to press hard enough to cause bruising or break any capillaries. Depending upon the thickness of the skin, work ten to twenty minutes on a particular area. Ten minutes should be sufficient for the tummy, but twenty minutes may be more useful for the upper thighs and hips. Massage any time of the day, but it is best to wait at least two hours after eating. The most convenient time for most men is after the bath or shower, preferably one that includes a brisk body rub with a loofah friction mitt. A bath is relax ing and recommended because a massage benefits the most when relaxed. Massage will improve blood and lymph circulation and minimize the appearance of hard fatty lumps. Apply a moisturizing cream or oil to the area to be massaged, so that the hands can glide smoothly over the skin. Massage firmly using the thumb and four fingers to grip the skin and fatty layer beneath it. Then knead in small circular movements as though working with dough. Then massage across the skin using the base of the palm of the hand, working in long, sweeping strokes toward the heart. Alternately, try a special hand-held massager with an oil or lotion to avoid excessive friction and broken capillaries.

HEALTHY BREATHING

When tense, breathing is likely shallow and too quick. As a result, the body is not getting enough oxygen. Anxiety is a symptom of this lack of oxygen. The lungs will not expel carbon dioxide efficiently, which results in fatigue. This vicious self-perpetuating circle needs to be broken in order to feel better. Deep breathing can calm you down within minutes and will energize you. Make sure to do deep breathing exercises during a fitness routine; inhale and exhale entirely as much as possible, ideally at least three times per day. The male body needs oxygen to increase vitality and stimulate internal irrigation system.

Deep Breathing Exercise

- Wear loose clothing and lie down
- Exhale through the mouth for as long as you can
- Inhale through the mouth, to a count of ten, feeling the diaphragm and the abdomen rise
- Try to inhale enough air to fill your lungs completely
- Slowly exhale to a count of twenty, pushing every breath of air from the lungs
- Try this for two or three minutes

GET MOVING

A comprehensive fitness plan should include the basics of flexibility, strength training, endurance, and aerobics. To stick with a healthy exercise routine, keep equipment in clear view and accessible, or join a gym that is in close proximity to your home or office, or hire a trainer to come to your home. Just keep it simple.

Exercising for the sole purpose of losing weight usually does not work. It is like doing a job that you hate or find unsatisfying just to get the paycheck. You may tolerate it for a while, but eventually you will give it up. You are more apt to persist if you are doing it for "internal" reasons such as feeling stronger or gaining confidence, rather than for purely "external" reasons. If you are going to stick with your workouts, they must make you feel good or give you a sense of accomplishment. A balanced fitness regimen should include some form of walking, treadmill, weights, and enough variations to make it interesting and enjoyable.

CONCLUSION

Male grooming has become a fact of life. Those who do not spend a little time maintaining their appearance may get noticed for all the wrong reasons.

A man faces tremendous emotional and physical challenges as he gets older. Changes at home, at work, and within his body all affect a man's general health and well-being.

Men who seek out cosmetic surgery generally have a positive self-image, despite being focused on one or more aspects of their appearance. In fact, some men may even feel better about their overall appearance than those who are uninterested in cosmetic surgery at all. In my practice, we have found that our male patients are overwhelmingly satisfied with the results as indicated by post-operative surveys. The perceived benefits include a boost in self-confidence, a better sex life, improved interpersonal relationships, and an increased enjoyment of the good things in life.

The Experts

OZ GARCIA

Oz Garcia, Ph.D., is CEO of the successful health lifestyle consulting firm, *Personal Best Inc.*, which specializes in progressive nutrition and anti-aging solutions. A highly regarded nutritional counselor and life extension specialist, Dr. Garcia was twice voted best nutritionist by *New York Magazine*. He lectures on the most current breakthroughs in therapeutic power foods and also on state-of the-art supplements and drugs to slow down the aging process and bring people to their highest health potential. Dr. Garcia works with many top CEO's and celebrities and has been featured in *Vogue*, *The New York Times*, and *Sports Illustrated*, among other publications. Dr. Garcia is also the best selling author of *The Balance* and *The Healthy HighTech Body*, updated and released as *Look and Feel Fabulous Forever* (ReganBooks/HarperCollins, January, 2003).

HOWARD MURAD, MD

As a pharmacist, dermatologist, associate clinical professor of dermatology at UCLA, and author, Dr. Howard Murad is recognized as one of the world's leading authorities in skin health. After earning his degree at the Brooklyn College of Pharmacy, he attended the University of California at Irvine Medical School. He completed his rotating internship back in New York at Queens Hospital. Dr. Murad completed his dermatology residency at the Veteran's Administration Hospital at UCLA. Today, Dr. Murad is still devoted to his dermatology practice in Los Angeles and sees patients regularly, combining his inclusive health treatments in both the Murad Medical practice and the Murad Medical Spa, which is located within his Inclusive Wellness Center.

MARC LOWENBERG, DDS

Dr. Marc Lowenberg is one of New York City's premiere cosmetic dentists, and he has perfected the smiles of numerous celebrities and public figures. Dr. Lowenberg holds a B.A. in psychology from the American

University in Washington, D.C. He graduated from New York University, College of Dentistry, after which he was granted a general practice internship at Metropolitan Hospital in New York City. His practice, Lowenberg & Lituchy, has been profiled on a variety of television programs including, *Good Morning America* and *The View*, and has been featured in *The New York Times*, *Vogue*, *People* and *InStyle*, among other publications.

FREDERIC FEKKAI

Frédéric Fekkai has become one of the most celebrated names in beauty and hairstyling, working with the world's most beautiful women and Hollywood's brightest stars. Acclaimed for his individualistic, common sense approach, Frédéric has built a luxury brand synonymous with the best in hair care for women and men. Along the way, he has left an indelible mark on the beauty and fashion communities with his innovative styling, exclusive salons, and range of extraordinary products. In 2000, Frédéric published his first book, *Frédéric Fekkai: A Year of Style*, a unique guide offering advice for living life more beautifully—including a style note for each day of the year.

DAVID FINLEY

David Finley, personal trainer, is an advocate of the "Super Slow" method. David Finley works with private clients in the New York Metro area, and has trained many corporate executives, and physicians. He has also developed training programs for the elderly and post-rehab clients.

ALLEN GREENBAUM, MD

Allen Greenbaum attended Mt. Sinai School of Medicine. He completed his ophthalmolgy residency at Mt. Sinai Hospital where he is now a clinical instructor. He is in private practice in White Plains, NY. In addition to general ophthalmology, he has a special interest in refractive and cataract surgery.

Glossary

A

Abdominoplasty —Commonly known as a tummy tuck, is a surgical procedure to remove excess skin and fat from the middle and lower abdomen and to tighten the muscles of the abdominal wall.

Ablation—Vaporization of the most superficial layers of skin.

Abscess— A localized collection of pus usually infected and caused by bacteria.

Acne—A chronic skin condition characterized by an inflammatory eruption of the skin that occurs when a hair follicle gets plugged with sebum and dead cells. Rising hormone levels stimulate oil glands, which cause clogged pores and inflammation.

Actinic Keratosis—(Solar keratosis) a lesion that is dry, scaly, rough, and tan or pink caused by sun exposure, considered precancerous.

Adipose tissue—A complex fatty layer of adiposities connective tissue and neurovasculature.

Adjustable gastric banding—Also known as the lap band, a small, silicone ring is placed around the stomach near the esophagus to limit food intake, using a laparoscopic approach. It has a thin silicone tube extension that connects to a fill dome placed just under the abdominal skin. Sterile water is injected into the dome to increase or decrease the constriction caused by the ring.

Allergen—A substance that can cause allergic reaction.

Allograft—A graft from the same species as the recipient, as in human skin.

Alopecia—A condition of hair loss.

Alpha Hydroxy Acid—(AHA) A group of acids derived from foods such as fruit and milk, which can improve the texture of the skin by removing layers of dead cells and encouraging cell regeneration. There are many AHA's but the most common are Lactic Acid, Glycolic Acid, Pyruvic Acid, Tartaric Acid and Maleic Acid.

Anemia—A pathological deficiency in the oxygen-carrying component of the blood, measured in unit volume concentrations of hemoglobin, red blood cell volume, or red blood cell number.

Anti-inflammatory—A substance known to counteract inflammation or swelling.

Antioxidant—A substance designed to prevent a chemical reaction with oxygen, e.g. Vitamins C, E, A, grape seed, green tea.

Areola—The naturally dark round pigmented area that surrounds the projecting nipple.

Arnica Montana—A botanical derived from a mountain plant with antiseptic, astringent, antimicrobial and anti-inflammatory properties.

Autogenous—Reconstructive material originating from one's own tissues.

Autologous—Occurring naturally in a certain type of tissue of the body.

Axillae—(plural of axilla) The armpit or the cavity beneath the junction of the arm and shoulder.

B

Basal Cell Carcinoma—cancer of one of the innermost cells of the deeper epidermis of the skin.

Benzoyl Peroxide—An antibacterial ingredient commonly used to treat acne.

Beta Hydroxy Acid (Salicylic Acid)—A family of acids that enhance cell renewal, found naturally in willow bark.

Bicep—The large flexor muscle of the front of the upper arm and back of the upper leg.

Bioactive—Substances that achieve cosmetic results by some degree of physiological action e.g. fruit acids.

Bleaching Agents—Substances which slow down or block the production of melanin to lighten age spots and fade areas of hyperpigmentation; i.e. Hydroquinone, Kojic Acid, Azelaic Acid.

Body Mass Index (BMI)—A measure of body fat that is the ratio of the weight of the body in kilograms to the square of its height in meters. A body mass index that exceeds a value of 25 indicates overweight. BMI between 30 and 35 is considered obese; over 35 is severely obese; and over 40 is morbidly obese.

Botulinium Toxin—A naturally occurring toxin that is injected into facial muscles to temporarily paralyze them and eliminate expression lines of the face, around the eyes, and the neck.

Bromelain—A protease obtained from the juice of the pineapple.

Buccal fat pad—A pad of cheek fat lying lateral to the lips and below the cheek bone. It remains rather large and descends into the jowls after weight loss and aging.

Buttock Crease—Lower fold of the buttocks.

C

Cannulae—Long, thin hollow tubular instrument with side openings near one end and a connection to high pressure suction machine on the other which is used to extract fat by vigorous back and forth motion during liposuction.

Capillary—The smallest type of blood vessel in the body. Spider veins, for instance, are actually small capillaries commonly found on the face or legs.

Carbon Dioxide—Laser technology that can be used to resurface moderate to deep facial wrinkles, scars, and can also be used as a cutting tool.

Cauterize—To burn or sear abnormal tissue with a cautery or caustic instrument, such as a laser.

Cellulite—Deposits of fat, toxins and fluids trapped in pockets beneath the skin, more common in women.

Chemical Peel—A procedure in which a solution of varying strengths is applied to the entire face or to specific areas, such as around the mouth, to peel away the skin's top layers. Common peeling agents are Alpha Hydroxy Acid, Beta Hydroxy Acid, Trichloracetic Acid (TCA), and Phenol.

Circumferential—Completely around a surface, as in a belt excision around the lower abdomen.

Co Enzyme Q10—A renewal agent that stimulates natural cell energy production and regenerates vitamin E.

Collagen—A primary component of human skin that gives it resiliency, suppleness and tone, and breaks down with age due to muscle movement and environmental damage.

Comedones—Open (blackheads) and closed (whiteheads) formed when pores become clogged with oils and impurities.

Commissure—The area where two anatomic parts meet, as in the corner of the eye or the lips, typically referring to a fold or crease.

Corrugator—Muscle that is responsible for causing the glabellar or vertical lines that form between the eyebrows.

Cosmeceutical—A substance that falls between the classification of a drug and a cosmetic, i.e., non-prescription over-the-counter formulations that provide pharmaceutical benefits.

Cryosurgery—Surgery in which diseased or abnormal tissue (as a tumor or wart) is destroyed or removed by freezing (as by the use of liquid nitrogen).

D

Deep vein thrombosis—The presence of a blood clot within a deeply positioned vein of the lower trunk or legs.

Dermal fillers—A category of substances that are either injected or implanted to shape and form overlying tissue.

Dermatitis—An inflammatory condition of the skin that is characterized by itching and redness.

Dermatopathology—Pathology of the skin.

Dermis—The layer of skin composed of collagen and elastin, lying beneath the epidermis (outer layer) and above the subcutaneous layers.

Diabetes—An altered state of sugar metabolism due to insensitivity to (Type II) or lack of insulin hormone (Type I). Type II is common in obesity and leads to a variety of disorders of the cardiovascular system, nervous system and skin, now called the metabolic syndrome.

Digestion—The process of making food absorbable by dissolving it and breaking it down into simpler chemical compounds that occurs in the living body chiefly through the action of enzymes secreted into the alimentary canal.

Diode—Contact laser technology that cuts and coagulates tissue.

Drain—A plastic multiperforated tube, connected to a compressible vacuum bulb, which is placed under skin flaps for a week or two to collect blood and serum.

E

Ecchymosis—The passage of blood from ruptured blood vessels into subcutaneous tissue, marked by a purple discoloration of the skin.

Echinacea—A natural substance thought to boost the immune system, and to have anti-itching and soothing properties.

Eczema—A chronic skin condition in areas of the skin and scalp.

Edema—An abnormal excess accumulation of serous fluid in connective tissue, such as ankle swelling or in a serous cavity, such as pulmonary congestion.

Elastin—A protein that is similar to collagen and the chief constituent of elastic fibers, also used as a surface protective agent in cosmetics to alleviate dry skin.

Epidermis—The outermost layer of the skin containing a maturing layer of epithelial cells including melanocytes, which impart color.

Epinephrine—A compound isolated from the adrenal glands and used in medicine as a heart stimulant, vasoconstrictor, and bronchial relaxant.

Epithelialization—Regeneration of the epithelium or superficial layer of the skin, as occurs after laser resurfacing.

Erbium:YAG—A type of ablative laser that produces energy in a wavelength that penetrates the skin, is readily absorbed by water (a major component of tissue cells), and scatters the heat effects of the laser light.

Erythema—Redness of the skin, as in post laser or other resurfacing, etc.

Exfoliate—To remove dead surface skin cells.

Extrusion—The erosion of skin that allows an implant (chin, lip, breast, etc.) to become exposed.

F

Fascia—The sheet of firm connective tissue that covers muscles, sometimes used as a graft material.

Fat Embolus—Particles of fat that enter the bloodstream during surgery and then spread to the lungs.

Fibroblast—A cell from which connective tissue develops.

Filler—A category of substances that are either injected or implanted to shape and form overlying tissue. Common fillers are Bovine collagen, the patient's own fat or hyaluronic acid gel.

Follicle—A sheath that surrounds the root of the hair.

Forehead Lift—Also called a brow lift, pulls up droopy brows and upper lids, and improves wrinkling and vertical and horizontal frown lines.

Free Radicals—A destructive form of oxygen generated by each cell in the body that destroys cellular membranes.

Frontalis—The muscle that enables the brows to move up and down, and contributes to the formation of horizontal wrinkles of the forehead.

G

General Anesthesia—Commonly referred to as being asleep. A total loss of consciousness induced through inhalation of special gases by an anesthetist (nurse) or anesthesiologist (physician). Your breathing is usually controlled through a tube placed in your airway and you won't feel anything. Supplemental intravenous narcotics and local anesthesia reduce surgical site pain upon awakening.

Glabella—The area between the eyebrows in the center of the forehead where deep vertical lines and creases often develop.

Glaucoma—Any of a group of eye diseases characterized by abnormally high intraocular fluid pressure, damaged optic disk, hardening of the eyeball, and partial to complete loss of vision.

Glycerin—Used in moisturizers due to its water binding capabilities.

Glycolic acid— The most commonly used alpha hydroxyl acid, glycolic acid affects the newly forming keratin cells at the bottom of the stratum corneum causing the bulk of the stratum corneum to lift off and separate from the underlying skin.

Graft—A piece of tissue that is totally removed from one part of the body and transferred to another area of the body, as in fat, cartilage, bone, skin, etc.

Gynecomastia—Male breast enlargement

H

Hematoma—A localized accumulation of blood in the skin caused by a blood vessel wall rupture, possible complication of surgery that may have to be drained.

Hirsutism—Excessive growth of hair of normal or abnormal distribution.

Hyaluronic Acid—An acid found naturally in the body and helps retain the skin's natural moisture.

Hydrocortisone—A glucocorticoid that is a derivative of cortisone and is used in the treatment of rheumatoid arthritis.

Hydroquinone—A bleaching agent that slows down or blocks the production of melanin to lighten age spots and to fade dark spots and blotchiness.

Hyperpigmentation—Darkening of the skin through overproduction of melanin by melanocytes.

Hypertension—Abnormally high arterial blood pressure, common in obesity and leads to severe cardiovascular occlusive disease, kidney insufficiency, stroke and premature death.

Hypertrophic scar—A thickened, elevated and red scar that fails to reduce in size over several months.

Hypertrophy—Enlarged volume through gain in cellular size or number.

Hypoallergenic—A substance with a low chance of causing allergy or skin irritation.

Hypopigmentation—Reduction in the pigment cells in the skin resulting in skin lightening

I

Informed Consent—A process of educating a patient with a reasonably amount of information regarding their treatment, alternatives to that treatment and risks of adverse events and complications.

Inframammary Fold—The skin fold that lies at the base of the breast and above the abdomen. Sagging breasts drape over this fold.

Intense Pulsed Light—Intense pulsed light (IPL) is an intense light that differs from a laser by using light that is neither coherent nor of a single wavelength

Isolagen—Autologous filler fashioned from collagen from your own skin that is grown in a laboratory, processed and liquefied for later injection into wrinkles and folds.

J

Jowls—Bulging laxity along the jaw lines lateral to the chin.

K

Keloid—Enlarged, permanent and thickened scar formations that are more common in darker skin types, and often run in families.

Keratin—A surface protective agent with film-forming and moisturizing action.

Kojic Acid—Natural skin-lightening agent derived from a Japanese mushroom.

L

L-ascorbic Acid—The purest form of Vitamin C, which when applied topically is an antioxidant, anti-irritant, anti-inflammatory.

Lactic Acid—A component of the skin's natural moisturizing factor.

Lap Band Adjustable Gastric Banding—An inflatable plastic restrictive ring placed around the stomach that variably restricts food intake.

Laparoscopic Surgery—Operations performed within the abdominal cavity through multiple portals by means of a laparoscope and specially designed instruments.

Lateral Thigh—Part of the thigh situated at or extending to the side.

Laxity—The quality or state of being loose.

Lentigo—Benign tan or brown colored lesion on the skin from sun exposure.

Lidocaine—A local anesthetic (trade name Xylocaine) used topically on the skin and mucous membranes and injected under the skin.

Lipoatrophy—Loss of facial or body fat beneath the skin, common in HIV patients

Local Anesthesia—Medications (usually in the 'caine' family) that are injected into a surgical or treatment site to cause temporary localized numbness.

Lymphatic System—A network of structures, including ducts and nodes that carry lymph fluid from tissues to the bloodstream.

M

Marionette Lines—The vertical creases that form in the corners of the mouth towards the jowls.

Melanin—The pigment that gives skin and hair its color.

Melanocytes—Cells which contain and produce melanin.

Melanoma—The deadliest form of skin cancer characterized by a black or dark brown pigmented tumor.

Mentalis—A muscle that originates on the mandible and inserts in the skin of the chin, and raises the chin. It pulls down the lower lip.

Microabrasion—A tooth-whitening procedure using an abrasive combined with a hydrochloric acid.

Microdermabrasion—A mechanical blasting of the face with sterile microparticles that abrade or rub off the very top skin layer, then vacuuming out the particles and the dead skin.

Milia—Tiny skin cysts that resemble whiteheads.

Mohs Surgery—The destruction of malignant, infected, or gangrenous tissue by the application of chemicals to remove skin cancers.

Monitored Anesthesia Care (MAC)—Also called 'local with intravenous sedation' and 'twilight sleep', where medications are given intravenously to induce a state of sleepiness and relieve pain, supplemented with local anesthetic injections.

Musculature—The system or arrangement of muscles in a body or a body part.

N

Nasolabial Folds—The region of the face between the nose and the corners of the lip, commonly referred to as 'smile lines'.

Nasion—The depression at the root of the nose that indicates the junction where the forehead ends and the bridge of the nose begins.

Necrosis—Dead or dying tissue.

Non-Ablative Laser Resurfacing—A category of lasers that do not produce a deep burn.

Non-comedogenic—Products that are formulated not to clog the pores and cause pimples.

O

Obesity—A condition characterized by excessive body fat and directly related chronic metabolic disorders such as diabetes.

Off-Label Use—The prescribed use of a drug or medical devise by a medical practitioner for an indication not approved by the Federal Drug Administration.

Orbicularis Oculi—The muscular body of the eyelid encircling the eye and comprising the palpebral, orbital, and lacrimal muscles. The palpebral muscle functions to close the eyelid gently; the orbital muscle functions to close it more energetically, such as in winking.

Orbit—The cavity in the skull where the eyeballs, eye muscles, nerves and blood vessels rest.

Outpatient Surgery—Ambulatory surgery in which you are discharged later the same day from the recovery room in a hospital, office surgical suite, or clinic.

P

Panniculectomy—Surgical excision of redundant pannus or section of skin and fat of the abdomen.

Parasternal—Near the junction of the sternum (breast plate) and the ribs.

Pectoralis Major Muscle—A large flat muscle immediately under the breast that extends from the first seven ribs to the upper arm humerus bone.

Periareolar—Refers to a circle around the areola.

Petrolatum—Used in creams, it softens and soothes skin. Forms a film to prevent moisture loss.

Ph—The degree of acidity or alkalinity in the solution of products.

Phlebitis—Inflammation of a vein.

Photoaging—Damage to the skin due to cumulative exposure to the sun; i.e. wrinkles, age spots, fine lines.

Photosensitivity—Chemicals or topical ingredients that cause the skin to be reactive when exposed to sunlight.

Platysma—A thin sheet of muscle located just beneath the skin of the chin and neck.

Platysmal Bands—Vertical strands of the muscle of the neck that can become more prominent with age and are often sutured or tightened during a face or neck lift.

Pore—Small opening of the sweat glands of the skin.

Procerus—Muscle that works with the corrugator muscles and contributes to the vertical frown lines between the eyebrows.

Psoriasis—An inflammatory skin condition characterized by recurring reddish patches covered with silvery scales.

Ptosis—Relating to or affected with the sagging of a structure or an organ.

Pulmonary Embolus—A blockage of an artery in the lungs by fat, air, tumor tissue, or blood clot.

R

Resorcinol—Used as an antiseptic and as a soothing preparation for itchy skin.

Retin-A™ (Tretinoin)—A topical medication derived from Vitamin A that is used to treat photoaging and acne.

Retinol—A non-prescription strength alternative to Retinoic Acid. Retinol is an active form of Vitamin A that works deep under the surface of the skin to reduce lines and wrinkles.

Rhytidectomy (Facelift)—Surgical procedure which rejuvenates the face by tightening the underlying musculature, removing excess fat deposits, and redraping sagging skin of the lower face and neck. Incisions are placed in the hairline and around the ears and/or under the chin.

Rosacea—A common skin condition of the face, nose, cheeks, forehead that results in redness, pimples, dilated blood vessels and occasional pustules.

S

Schirmer's Test—A test that assesses tear production in the eyes and is helpful in treating dry eye syndrome.

Sclerotherapy—The injection of one of several solutions through a small needle directly into a vein to cause it to collapse.

Sebborheic Keratoses—Benign lesions on the surface of the skin that don't turn into cancer.

Septoplasty—An operation to straighten a crooked (deviated) septum in order to improve breathing.

Septum—The separating wall in the nose between the left and right nasal passages.

Seroma—A pool of clear fluid called serum lying under the skin most often following operations that leave large spaces such as flap and liposuction surgery.

SFS—An acronym for Superficial Fascial System. It is a multilayered organized collagenous layer of the subcutaneous tissue that is carefully preserved and sutured together under tension during body-contouring surgery.

Silastic sheeting—Patches or strips of silicone that may be applied to the skin for extended time periods to soften and reduce scarring.

Silicone—A synthetic substance used in a gel-like form in silicone breast implants, in a liquid injectable form for facial areas, and in other medical devices.

Sleep apnea—Intermittent periods of brief cessation of breathing during sleep. It is caused in the obese by obstruction of the airway and is associated with excessive daytime sleepiness and irritability. When chronic and severe it leads to pulmonary hypertension, congestive heart failure and even death.

SMAS—an acronym for Superficial Musculo Aponeurotic System. It is a firm layer of tissue that covers the superficial muscles in the cheek and extends over the lower face and neck muscle called the platysma.

SPF (Sun Protection Factor)—A scale used to rate the level of protection sunscreens provide from UVB rays of the sun.

Spider Veins (Telangiectasias)—Dilated or broken blood vessels near the surface of the skin.

Squamous Cell Carcinoma—The second most common skin cancer that arises from the epidermis and resembles the squamous cells that comprise most of the upper layers of skin.

Sternal Notch—The top of the sternum at the midline base of the neck between the collarbones.

Steroids—Any of a large number of hormonal substances with similar basic chemical structure, produced mainly in the adrenal cortex and gonads.

Stratum Corneum—Surface layer of epidermis.

Striae—Commonly known as stretch marks, cause by thinning of the underlying skin layer (dermis) and rupture of elastic fibers that appear first as red, raised lines, then darken and flatten gradually to form shiny whitened streaks.

Subcutaneous Tissue—The variably thick composite connective and adipose tissue between the skin and muscular fascia. The adipose imparts skins softness, pliability, surface contour and body warmth and protection.

Suction Assisted Lipectomy (Liposuction)—A procedure in which localized collections of fat are removed from the face and/or body by using a high vacuum device through small incisions.

Sun Block—A physical sunscreen or a barrier against the sun's ultraviolet rays.

Suture—A strand or fiber used to sew together parts of the living body. Permanent sutures do not dissolve and absorbable sutures do disappear in time.

T

T-Zone—The area of the face that consists of the forehead, nose and the area around the mouth, including the chin.

Tartaric Acid—A type of glycolic acid derived from apples.

Tazarotene—A prescription topical retinoid (vitamin A derivative) approved for treating mild to moderate plaque psoriasis and photo aging.

Tissue Engineering—The science of production of human tissue ex vivo, (outside of the human body) as in growing cartilage in tissue culture.

Titanium Dioxide—A non-chemical, common agent used in sunscreen products that works by physically blocking the sun. It may be used alone or in combination with other agents.

Tretinoin—A derivative of vitamin A.

Trichloroacetic Acid—A colorless compound, used topically as an astringent, antiseptic, and skin peeling agent.

Tumescent—A method of anesthesia where large volumes of local anesthetic and saline solution are injected to swell the area to be operated on, commonly used in liposuction and body contouring procedures.

Tumescent Infiltration—A method to provide tissue numbness and decrease bleeding prior to incisions and liposuction. Small amounts of xylocaine for local anesthesia and epinephrine for vasoconstriction are added to large volumes of saline which is then infiltrated into the operative regions until the tissues are sufficiently swollen.

U

Ultrasound—Application of a sound wave, a mechanical vibration of more than 16,000 cycles per second.

UVA—Long wavelengths emitted by the sun which take longer to produce a burn than UVB but penetrate deeper into the skin to cause sun damage.

UVB—Short wavelengths emitted by the sun, which are known to cause premature aging and skin cancer.

Umbilicus—Belly button or navel.

V

Varicose Veins—Enlarged, swollen and dilated veins just below the surface of the skin, commonly found in the legs and caused by the valves becoming filled with blood.

W

Wavelength—The distance between a given point on one wave cycle and the corresponding point on the next successive wave cycle.

X

Xanthoma—A fatty deposit in the skin that may appear on the lower eyelids or elsewhere.

Y

YAG—Abbreviation for yttrium aluminum garnet, a crystal used in some types of lasers.

Z

Zinc Oxide—Chemical ingredient that has soothing and astringent qualities that can block ultraviolet rays of the sun.

Index

P

Panniculectomy, 63, 197
Parasternal, 197
Pectoralis Major Muscle, 53, 60, 198
Periareolar, 198
pH, 104, 106
Phlebitis, 198
Photoaging, 14-5, 198
Photosensitivity, 198
Platysma, 198-99
Platysmal Bands, 198
Polysaccharide, 45
Pore, 15, 70-5, 83, 89, 93, 118, 120, 128, 189, 191, 197-98
Procerus, 198
Psoriasis, 78, 81-2, 198, 200
Ptosis, 198
Pulmonary Embolus, 198

R

Retin-A (Tretinoin), 76, 113, 122, 198, 200
Retinol, 198
Rhytidectomy, 198
Rosacea, 77-8, 199

S

Schirmer's Test, 199
Sclerotherapy, 199
Sebborheic Keratoses, 199
Septoplasty, 199
Septum, 39-40, 180, 199
Seroma, 61, 63, 199
SFS, 67, 199
Silicone, 36, 38, 43, 51, 59-60, 64, 104-05, 189, 199
Sleep apnea, 65, 179-80, 199
SMAS, 199
SPF, 71,

Spider Veins, 191, 199
Squamous Cell Carcinoma, 94, 98-9, 200
Sternal Notch, 200
Subcutaneous Tissue, 45, 192, 199-200
Steroids, 54, 79-80, 82, 116, 118, 122, 200
Stratum Corneum, 194, 200
Suction Assisted Lipectomy, 200
Sun Block, 34, 92-3, 130, 200
Suture, 25, 31, 37, 39, 49, 57, 60, 67, 198-200

T

Tazarotene, 76, 82, 200
Tissue Engineering, 200
Titanium Dioxide, 92, 200
Tretinoin, 76, 113, 198, 200
Trichloroacetic acid, 191, 201
Tumescent, 56, 201

U

Ultrasound, 62, 67, 124, 201
UVA, 82, 92-3, 201
UVB, 34, 82, 92-3, 199, 201
Umbilicus, 63, 201

V

Varicose Veins, 135-36, 159, 201

X

Xanthoma, 201

Y

YAG, 127, 193, 201

Z

Zinc Oxide, 92, 201

Notes